Train your Bacl

For my parents

Alexander Jordan

Train Your Back

Versatile Exercises for a Healthy Back

Meyer & Meyer Sports

Original title: Rückentraining
- Aachen: Meyer & Meyer Verlag, 2001
Translated by Heather Ross

British Library Cataloguing in Publication Data
A catalogue record for this book is available from the British Library

Jordan, Alexander:
Train your Back/Alexander Jordan
Oxford: Meyer & Meyer Sport (UK) Ltd., 2002
ISBN 1-84126-073-8

© 2002 by Meyer & Meyer Sport (UK) Ltd.
Aachen, Adelaide, Auckland, Budapest, Graz, Johannesburg,
Miami, Olten (CH), Oxford, Singapore, Toronto
Member of the World
Sports Publishers' Association (WSPA)
www.w-s-p-a.org

Printed and bound in Germany
by: Druckpunkt Offset GmbH, Bergheim
ISBN 1-84126-073-8
E-Mail: verlag@meyer-meyer-sports.com
www.meyer-meyer-sports.com

Contents

Foreword

It appears to be a function of modern life that an increasing number of people seem to have serious health problems. Restricted movement, resulting in muscular tension, stress and other mental disorders are having a negative effect on personal wellbeing. Many of these health problems seem to focus on the back and the lower back in particular. Different patterns of work and a society where work, family and leisure are undergoing change, as well as an ever-changing environment are having a negative effect on us. The question is what to do about it? The important thing is that you act as soon as possible because prevention is always more pleasant, pain free and cheaper than cure.

As more and more people realise this they are becoming increasingly interested in exercise, sports and other leisure activities, making lifestyle changes that will bring about positive benefits to their individual health and wellbeing. In fact a well-planned and correctly implemented health and fitness training programme adopted as part of a daily routine can improve both health and the feeling of wellbeing.

Well-balanced exercise plays an important role here and the systematic strengthening and stretching of individual muscle groups will improve joint stability without decreasing mobility. If you add to this that this type of training can provide the necessary motivation to encourage the individuals to continue and develop then you have a winning formula.

This book provides an exercise programme that should improve the fitness of even the most "aching" back. It provides ideas for exercises that can be done at home as well as at a gym. It provides a blueprint for a gentle individual pain relieving programme as well as ideas for pair work and for using equipment.

At this point I may express a couple of personal ideas.

Firstly, in this book I have had the opportunity to work on a project that has been close to my heart for many years. Inspired by the Dance Exercise presented by Gundula Otta in Göttingen, I had the opportunity to develop further studies which permitted me to offer a series of courses for such as high schools, sports clubs and other public bodies. I also worked on the development of a professional qualification in Exercise Leadership. In this book I would like to pass on to you the experience that I have gained during many years of work. In this way I hope to motivate you, as I have managed to do with many others, to exercise regularly and above all to look after your back.

Secondly, this book also follows the principles of Natascha and Martin Hillebrecht. I would also like to pass on my grateful thanks to those whose commitment and support help me to produce my work. These include the models, Sonja Weiland and Bastian Bodecker, whose patience and skill resulted in the many illustrations that accompany each exercise. Additionally, to Rudolf Hillebrecht, who has proved an outstanding and completely reliable photographer. Finally, I would like to express my thanks to those who stood on the sidelines and worked in the background on the production of this book.

I wish all my readers a great deal of fun in practice and training and hope that you will be stimulated by the ideas presented.

Alexander Jordan

For those readers unfamiliar with anatomical terminology the following are used in this book:

Cervical spine = *the neck region of the spine*

Thoracic spine = *the region of the spine around the ribs*

Lumbar spine = *the lower back around the hip area*

The Sternum = *the breast bone*

Ischium = *the bone you "sit on"*

Proprioception = *the ability to know exactly where any part of the body is in space at any given time*

Gluteous muscles (maximus, medius and minimus) = *the muscles of the bottom*

Quadriceps = *the muscle in front of the thigh*

Throughout this book, the pronouns he, she, him, her and so on are interchangeable and intended to be inclusive of both men and women. It is important in sport, as elsewhere, that men and women have equal status and opportunities.

A BASIC INFORMATION

▬ Basic principles of training for a healthy back
▬ The teaching principles that underlie effective training for a healthy back
▬ Understanding the exercises
▬ Preparation to exercise

▯ Developing a Healthy Lifestyle through Training Your Back

Focus

In this chapter a rationale will be presented to justify the exercises selected. How important is it to train the back? What are its advantages? What are the potential dangers, and above all a health and fitness perspective is provided. In the second part a method of which to choose and how to do the exercises is suggested. By practically performing the exercises it will appreciated exactly how and why they fit together.

1 Help Your Back - Feel Healthy

Back trouble, Back pain?! Unfortunately, more than three quarters of all individuals know this problem only too well. A changing environment with fewer and fewer possibilities for movement is probably the main, but not the only, cause The problem is complex, and there often seems to be no way out. The spine is turning out to be the weakest point of the human skeleton.

The spine constitutes the main organ that enables one to stand upright. It gives us many possibilities, but also adopts several functions. The spine consists of vertebrae and discs, like a series of building bricks and sponges placed alternately on top of each other. It can simultaneously provide high mobility and static durability. The spine can thus bend and stretch (straighten), it can hyperextend and turn, twist and bend to the side - individually, one movement at a time, as well as different combinations.

9

This variety of movement of the spine as a chain of joints assures tension in the muscle system. If the muscles function correctly, the spine can accomplish its tasks. However, the muscles in particular tend either to loosen or shorten as a result of defective movements. If this happens often enough, the vertebrae and thus the spine can no longer move and protect properly. This leads to so-called slipped disc and overloading, and the pain that results from this.

The back training presented here deals with this deficiency: in order to prevent muscle weakening and shortening, regular strengthening and stretching exercises must be performed in order to train the muscles surrounding the spine.

However, this is only part of the problem, for modern thinking on health advocates turning right away from high risk factors to a more educational approach. So a concern for the development of personal protection factors is the priority. Back training consisting only of strength training and stretching would only deal with part of this concept, namely the development of physical protection factors in the form of improved fitness. However, the complete (holistic) consideration of a person's social, professional, economic and ecological living conditions seems to be far more important, as they create a predominant feeling for life, which can then be assessed separately as healthy or unhealthy.

The educational objective of sports teaching in schools and sports suppliers in clubs is legitimized in part by the promotion of the health of the pupils and participants. That is why the planning of supplies in sports education like back training in particular should follow holistic objectives, which are reflected in the selection of the following contents and methods.

2 The Structure of Exercise - the Principles of Exercise Prescription

Movement and sporting activities are rarely sufficient by themselves and develop further only conditionally. For functional gymnastic activities, such as back training, it is even truer than for team sports, for instance. If modern awareness of movement and training theory and sports medicine and sports psychology is used, then it must be incorporated into the gymnastics exercises. It gives rise to a pedagogical teaching situation. The basis of education rests on the idea of transmitting a didactic conception of the organisation of the teaching and learning process (figure 1). Exercises and training as learning phases are included in this.

Back Training

Approach

Aimed at preventive protection via movement and training of the back, to improve health and increase fitness.

Continuity – Regularity – Planning

At work – In the club – In the gym

Goals

Physiological Goals	Cognitive goals	Affective-emotional goals	Social goals
• Prevention against back pain • Strengthening the supporting muscles • Improving the mobility of the spine	• Knowledge of anatomical-physiological basics • Knowledge of correct back posture • Health provision	• Promotion of joyful movement • Improvement of proprioception and relaxation • Development of self-confidence • Increased happiness	• Promotion of sociability • Development of conversation and contacts • Strengthening of links • Partner and group exercises

Contents

Topics

• Warming up
• Muscle strengthening
• Joint stabilizing
• Proprioception
• Games and playing
• Relaxation

Equipment

• Exercise bar
• Exercise band
• Swiss ball
• ...

Methods

• Learning the starting positions and basic postures
• Getting to know the exercise principles with the help of selected exercises
• Guidance in the principles:
  – from known to unknown
  – from easy to hard
  – from simple to complex

• Correcting each other
• Partner: from passive-supporting to an active-exercising pair work.

Development of a healthy Lifestyle

Arousing, experiencing and forming health in its entirety in the subjective-individual wellbeing, and thereby developing a self-determined and responsible personality

Figure 1: Didactics of back training

11

Prerequisites - starting points

Nothing comes from nothing! So take your decision to begin goal-oriented, preventive back training seriously. Have the courage to take yourself in hand and carry out your exercise programme regularly. Naturally, training should be fun and above all, you should feel good afterwards. But to begin with, this is important: start today! Maybe you can encourage friends and acquaintances to participate, the more the merrier!

Developing a healthy lifestyle

Lifestyle is the sum of many, often competing, factors from which an individual has to choose. These include factors from the work, education, home and social environments. It is important to remember that even fashion and trends can have an impact on lifestyle. Never forget that lifestyle selection is a very personal thing which the individual must be allowed to choose for themselves. Because the competing influences are very strong it is by no means certain that the correct decision will be made, and each individual must bear in mind previous decisions and review the impact that they have had on lifestyle.

Once someone has selected a healthy lifestyle they should be encouraged to continue to maintain it, and the back exercises promoted in this book should do just this. Sport and exercise are only two means of training, both of which can provide tangible effects for certain people. Because of the social nature of sport, for example, it is possible to establish and maintain meaningful relationships with a variety of different people, which can range from informal casual acquaintances to deep and lasting friendships. In addition to such social benefits the individual gains a balanced approach to life which can have an impact on body image and hence indirectly personality.

❚❚❚ Training Tips – What You Should Always Bear in Mind

Focus

In this chapter, you can read how to work with the practical part of the book. Above all you will receive guidelines on how to understand the exercise descriptions. There are also hints and tips as to how to put together your own training programme from these exercises, and what you should watch out for, when you are exercising at home. In the practical section "Proprioception - Awareness of Spinal Posture" and "Correct Starting Positions for the Exercises", you will learn the essential principles for the correct reproduction of the exercises. Practise the individual exercise starting positions; they are the basis of the exercises that follow.

1 The Exercises

The practical exercises form the core of this book. They constitute your extensive and varied training programme. They work and develop your back. Your muscle strength, your flexibility, your posture and your coordination will be improved.

Which different exercise areas (chapters) are there?

The exercises are separated into different areas. These areas comprise both exercises without equipment for stretching and strengthening and for improving flexibility, and strengthening exercises with an exercise bar. Finally, there are relaxation exercises. The exercises are subdivided into specific areas of the body; beginning with the chest-shoulder-arms area and ending with the legs.

The transitions between the separate areas are fluid, however. First of all, go to the exercise focus, where in each case you can read the formulated training goal of the exercise.

So that you may clarify the position and names of the muscles grouped in the exercise areas which form the important training aims, please see the following illustrations.

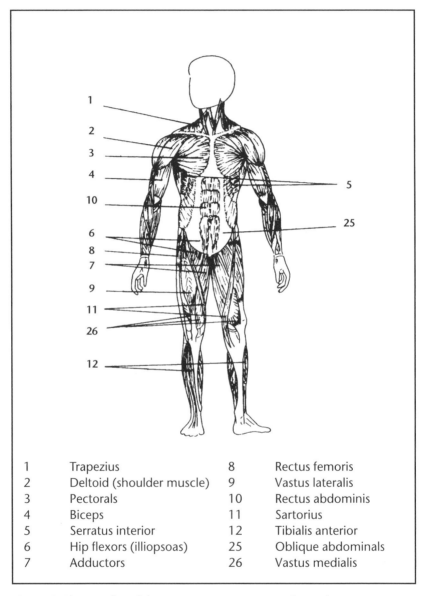

1	Trapezius	8	Rectus femoris
2	Deltoid (shoulder muscle)	9	Vastus lateralis
3	Pectorals	10	Rectus abdominis
4	Biceps	11	Sartorius
5	Serratus interior	12	Tibialis anterior
6	Hip flexors (illiopsoas)	25	Oblique abdominals
7	Adductors	26	Vastus medialis

Figure 2: The muscles of the movement apparatus – front view
(illustration modified after MEDLER/MIELKE 1994, 20)

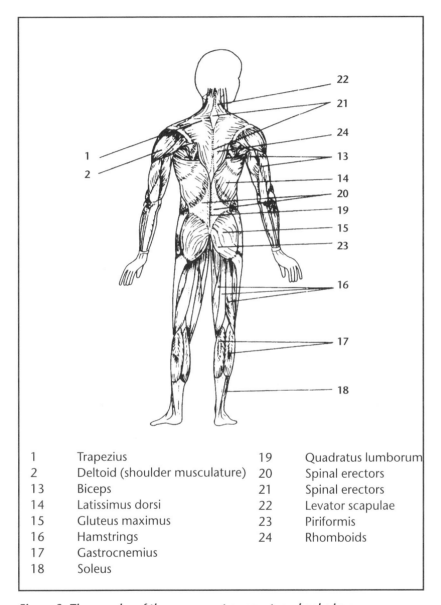

1	Trapezius	19	Quadratus lumborum
2	Deltoid (shoulder musculature)	20	Spinal erectors
13	Biceps	21	Spinal erectors
14	Latissimus dorsi	22	Levator scapulae
15	Gluteus maximus	23	Piriformis
16	Hamstrings	24	Rhomboids
17	Gastrocnemius		
18	Soleus		

Figure 3: The muscles of the movement apparatus – back view
(illustration modified after MEDLER/MIELKE 1994, 21)

15

Which system are the exercise descriptions based on?
The exercises are described according to a general system, which should facilitate your understanding of the exercise procedures.

- **Numbering and naming:** The exercises are numbered continuously. The names are given again according to the basic organisation of the exercises in the table of contents, and further designated special conditions such as the use of equipment or exercises with a partner.
- **Training goal:** Here you can learn the main purpose of the exercises. The explanations of muscular and coordinative effects also appear.
- **Description:** Find out the starting positions and movements for each exercise. The descriptions of the starting position refer to the adoption of an exercise posture in the correct starting positions for the exercises described in this chapter. Then the exercises are illustrated with at least one photograph. Photos without a subtitle refer to how the described exercise should be carried out.
- **Tip:** To avoid mistakes, to correct yourself, or to gain additional knowledge, you will find here more in-depth information on the exercise descriptions. You should pay special attention to the comments on "points of awareness".
- **Variations:** You receive suggestions as to how to vary the exercises. You thereby avoid possible monotony and can vary both the intensity and the difficulty of the exercises. Some exercise variations are also illustrated with photos. Just compare the subtitle with the number of the variation.
- **Partner work:** In pair-work exercises, additional guidelines on each basic position will be given, in which both partners work together. Three possibilities will be given:
    a. one partner carries out the exercise, the other assists, supports, reinforces or makes the exercise more difficult.
    b. Both partners carry out different exercises.
    c. Both partners carry out the same exercise together.

The further exercise descriptions also vary, dependent on the exercise situation. So, for example, in the second possibility, the training goals will be different for each partner.

2 Level of Difficulty of the Exercise

The strengthening exercises in the practical section are explained additionally according to the given system of exercise-specific degree of difficulty.

On which criteria are the degrees of difficulty based?
Each exercise is assessed according to its conditioning and coordination prerequisites as well as its movement complexity, and graded by category: "easy", "medium" and "hard".

What information does the degree of difficulty give?
The degree of difficulty gives useful information which facilitates the comparison of the exercises:
■ which level of fitness you should have to carry out the exercise correctly
■ how to organise the exercises to achieve the desired training effects
■ they are structured in an order you should follow when carrying out the individual exercises. You should work on the principle "from easy to hard".

How is an individual stretching and strengthening programme put together?
Check the degree of difficulty of your choice of exercise. Combine the exercises according to your individual wishes and goals and focus on your individual exercise emphasis. You can also use the possibilities of the short programmes:
■ Take one of the short programmes, according to the training emphasis. You should determine which exercises don't suit you or do not load enough, simply exchange these exercises for others. The degree of difficulty can help you in this. Be careful that the exercises replace the same function area.
■ Make sure you warm up before the exercises and relax afterwards.

3 Correct Starting Positions for the Exercises

Learn the principles of a correct starting position for each body position for the exercises. They are the basis for the exercises in the training programme.

1 Basic supine position

Description

Starting position: Lie on your back on the floor. Bend your knees at right-angles, hip width apart, until the soles of the feet can touch the floor.
The arms are slightly bent at the elbows and lie on the floor next to the body, the palms of the hands face upwards.

Basic Tension: Flex both feet and push your heels into the floor.
Keep your lumbar spine in contact with the floor, buttock and stomach muscles brace, your shoulder blades move towards each other.
Your arms and hands press against the floor, your cervical spine stretches right back.

Exercise: *Lift your head and shoulder girdle from the floor.*
Raise your arms slightly from the floor, the wrists bent slightly outwards.
Keep your cervical spine stretched throughout. Look up.

Tips

▪ Don't bring your head towards your chest.
To vary the load on the cervical spine musculature, put your hands behind your head. Your hands support the head, and the elbows stick right out to the sides.
▪ Keep the tension in the buttock muscles, so that the lumbar spine remains in contact with the floor. Make this easier by pulling in your feet.

Variations

a. As described, lift your head and shoulder girdle and press your lower arms and hands hard onto the floor.

b. As described in variation a., in addition, pull the knees at a right angle alternately to the stomach.

c. As described in variation b, in addition, press with the same-sided hand on the outside or front of the pulled-in knee. Keep the basic tension with your other arm and leg.

d. As described in variation b, press both hands against the knees pulled into the stomach. Keep your knees hip width apart.

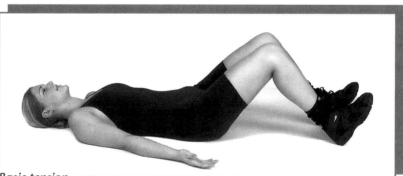

Basic tension

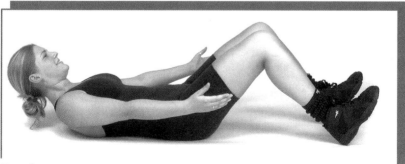

Exercise

19

2 Basic prone position

Description

Starting position: Lie in the prone position on the floor.
Your feet are hip width apart with the arches of your feet out. Your arms lie in the u-position with the palms of the hands on the floor, the fingers pointing forwards. Your elbows are bent at right-angles, your upper arms are in line with your shoulder girdle.Your forehead lies on the floor, pull your chin towards your chest.

Basic tension: Flex your feet as far as possible, the tips of your toes stay on the floor.
Keep your legs straight.
Tilt your pelvis by tensing your gluteus maximus muscles. At the same time, press your pubic bone against the floor, lift your iliac crest from the floor, your navel is raised slightly from the floor. Your lumbar spine is flat throughout. Press your arms and hands from the elbows up to the palm of the hands onto the floor.

Exercise: Lift your hands and arms from the floor, the palms of your hands facing each other, the thumbs pointing upwards. The shoulder blades move towards each other.

Tips
- Hold the basic tension consciously through the lumbar spine and pelvis. The straightening of the lumbar spine is only possible if the lower trunk musculature is well-tensed.
- Establish the basic tension with gentle and regular breathing. Breathe out when tensing, breath in when relaxing.

20

Variations

a. As described, but raise only one arm, while pressing the other arm down hard on the floor.
b. As described in variation a., straightening your arms.
c. As described in variation b., take your arms alternately backwards down the sides, and then forwards again.

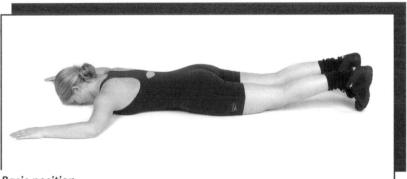

Basic position

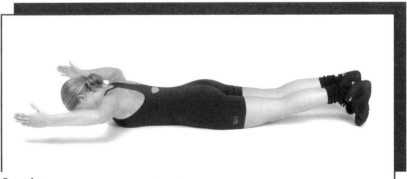

Exercise

3 Basic side position

Description

Starting position: Lie on your side on the floor.
Your legs are placed on top of each other, so that your head, your pelvis and your heels are in a straight line. Keep your pelvis poised perpendicularly. Your top arm is placed on the floor in front of your chest. Your head lies on your bottom arm in line with your spine.

Basic tension: Flex both feet.
Raise your upper leg to hip-height.
Tense your buttock and stomach muscles in order to fix your lumbar spine. Press down on the floor with your supporting hand.

Tips
■ Keep your legs absolutely still.
■ Maintain the tension between your shoulder blades.

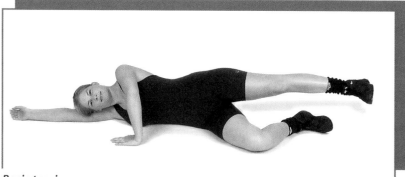

Basic tension

4 Basic kneeling position

Description

Starting Position: Kneel with your legs hip width apart on the floor. The arches of your feet are laid out on the floor. Straighten your spine from the pelvis upwards up through the thoracic and cervical spine. Your sternum is pushed forwards and upwards, while your shoulders drop downwards and backwards. Keep your head in line with your spine.

Basic Tension: Tense the muscles of your trunk firmly, especially your stomach and buttock muscles. Place your fingers behind your head and press them hard against your head. Your elbows stick right out to the side. Maintain the tension in your trunk.

Tip

■■ Don't push your upper body and head forwards with your hands.

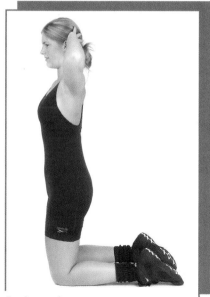

Basic tension

5 Basic "all fours" position

Description

Starting Position: Get onto all fours on the floor, with your knees hip-width apart below your hip joints, your thighs perpendicular and the arches of your feet on the floor. Place your hands under your shoulders, with your fingers pointing slightly diagonally inwards, your elbows slightly bent. Extend your cervical spine in line with your spine, at the same time pushing the back of your head away from the centre of the body, and pull your chin slightly towards your neck.

Basic tension: Pull in your feet, keeping the tips of your toes on the floor. Tense your stomach and buttock muscles. Press down with your hands on the floor and maintain the increasing tension between your shoulder blades.

Exercise: Extend one leg horizontally backwards, keeping your foot bent throughout.

Tips
- Distribute your bodyweight evenly on both hands.
- Keep the natural curves of your spine.
- Before going on all fours, first of all stretch your wrists. This prevents you feeling pain prematurely when carrying out the exercise.
- Do not use the alternative hand position, where you support yourself on your fists. This is an unstable position, and encourages a muscular imbalance in the lower arm, which is the source of wrist pain in the "all fours" position.

Variations:
a. As described, in addition, extend the opposite arm forwards to the leg extended backwards. Keep the palms of your hands flat on the floor.

24

Exercise situation: One partner carries out the exercise, the other controls it.

b. Adopt the "basic all fours" position. Your partner checks your position with an exercise bar, which he places on your back. Rest the pole on the back of your head and between your shoulder blades and on your coccyx. At the same time, your partner should place his fingers between the pole and your lumbar spine. This is the correct position for your spine.

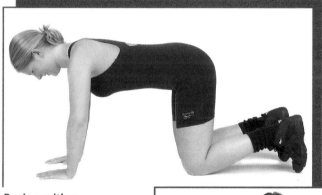

Basic position

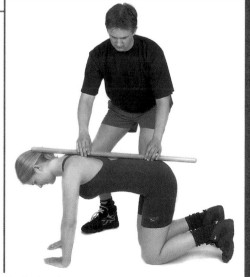

Variation b

25

6 Basic sitting position

Description

Starting Position: Sit on a chair.
The soles of your feet are placed flat and balanced on the floor. Your legs are bent at right angles at the knee and hip.
Align your feet and legs correctly. Your ankle, knee and hip joints are in one plane; an imaginary line runs down from your thigh above the middle toe.
Open your knees a little more than shoulder-width apart. Form an angle with your legs.
Tilt your pelvis forwards: and with a rocking movement of the pelvis forwards and backwards, hold the point at which the pressure on the ischium is clearly felt. This is the posture that results in the physiological posture of the lumbar spine. Lift your chest diagonally forwards and upwards.
Your shoulder girdle is relaxed; the shoulder blades move towards each other and pull slightly downwards. Your arms and hands are relaxed and lie on your thighs.
Extend your cervical spine; look straight ahead and perpendicular to the floor.

Basic tension: Press your feet down onto the floor and pull your heels in towards your body.
Grip your hands together in front of your chest and push your elbows right out to the sides.
Maintain your upright posture, particularly in your lower torso.

Tips
■ The described starting position provides an ideal body posture. You should use this as a model, while also endeavouring to find and practise your own individual posture- if necessary slightly different.

■ At first, try the movements of the different parts of the body and joints separately, before you finally try to adopt the upright sitting posture. Instead of a chair, you can also use a stool or a Swiss ball. Make sure that your hip joints are higher than your knee joints. Your thighs should slope slightly downwards and forwards. This will facilitate the tilting of the pelvis and also the straightening of the whole spine. If necessary, place a cushion on the seat of the chair.

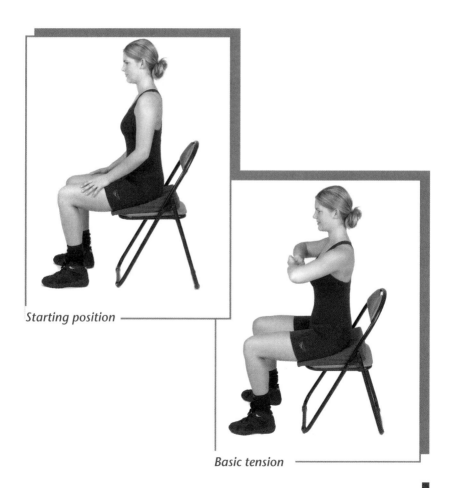

Starting position

Basic tension

7 Basic position - straight back, bent-over

Description

Starting position: Stand upright, feet hip-width apart, your feet pointing slightly outwards.
Transfer your centre of gravity downwards, bend your knees, your upper body remains perpendicular. Ensure that your leg posture is correct, so that foot, knee and hips are aligned.
Bend your upper body forward at the hips, your spine is firm, your cervical spine is in line with the rest of the spine.

Basic Tension: From this forward lean of your upper body, push your arms hard downwards and backwards in line with the side of the body and flex your wrists forwards.
Tense your trunk muscles.

Exercise: *Extend both arms alternately upwards and forwards.*

Tips
- If you want to adopt a straight-backed bent-over posture in order to lift heavy objects, you should carry out over the movement sequence described under "starting position from the upright position".
- Bend your knees maximally up to a right angle.
Do not relax the basic tension in your trunk; keep your spine stable.
- In the straight-backed bent-over posture, you can carry out functional strengthening exercises for your leg and back muscles.
- In your daily activities, remember to lift and carry heavy objects close to the body.

Variation
a. "Basic posture deep torso bend": bend your upper body from the straight-backed bent-over posture even further, maximally until it is horizontal, also keeping your cervical spine straight.

Now bring both straightened arms from their rear position forwards and upwards and then bend them. Keep your arms stable in the u-position, the palms of your hands perpendicular and your thumbs pointing upwards. Maintain the tension between your shoulder blades and in the upper trunk. Your lumbar spine is arched slightly forwards; it should never be rounded backwards.

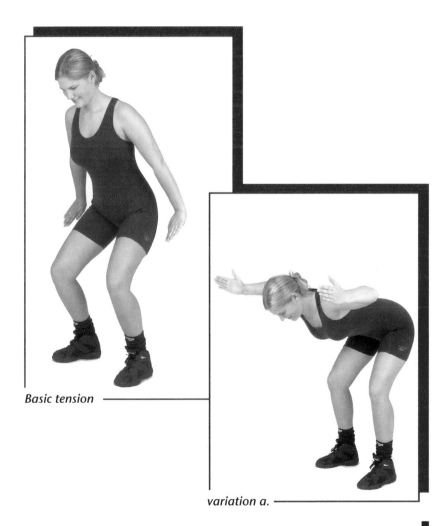

Basic tension ─────────

variation a. ─────────

29

8 Basic standing position

Description

Starting position: Stand with feet and legs hip-width apart, your feet pointing slightly outwards. Your knee joints are loose, under muscular tension, and are slightly bent. Your hips, knees and ankles are in line. Your pelvis is tilted, so that your spine can straighten physiologically. Straighten your chest, while pulling your sternum diagonally forwards and upwards.
Keep your head in line with your spine, look straight ahead. Your shoulder girdle is relaxed. Your arms hang relaxed down the sides of the body.
If you turn your arms slightly outwards, you support the extension of the spine; your shoulder blades are brought together.

Basic tension: Tense your buttock and stomach muscles. Stabilise your shoulder girdle by moving your shoulder blades together and downwards at the same time. Breathe calmly and regularly.

Tips
■ In order to take up the upright standing posture, pay special attention to lifting your chest and extending your cervical spine.
■ To control your posture, carry out the following exercise with your partner called "letting fall a perpendicular": Stand upright. Your partner tries to correct your posture by dropping a plummet from a sand bag ("heavy object") and a rope in profile down your side. The plummet should ideally pass down the middle of the ears, the shoulders, the pelvis and the feet. Your knees should remain slightly bent throughout.

■ It is vital for the exercise of the upright body posture while standing that you do not concentrate on the position of the spine, but that you interiorise the general idea of "standing".

■ From this ideal posture that your partner has helped you to correct, you must now develop your own individual posture. In any case, make sure that the upwards stretch of your body is maintained. You should feel comfortable in this posture.

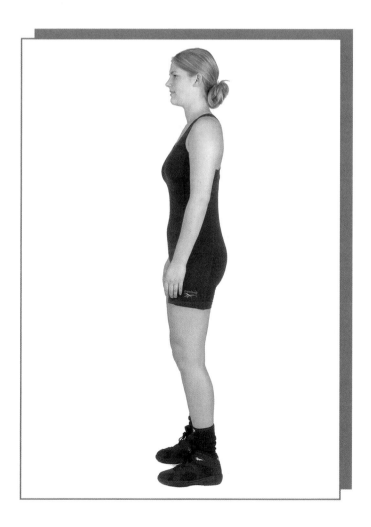

4 Proprioception
– Awareness of Spinal Posture

The following exercises form a sequence. Carry out the individual exercises one after the other, while being aware of the different positions of your spine.

9 Proprioception – awareness of spinal posture

TRAINING GOAL   **Awareness** of the position of the spine
                     Awareness of the separate vertebrae
                     Flexibility of the spine

Description
Starting position: Adopt the "Basic Prone Position".
Exercise: Rock your pelvis backwards and forwards, be aware of the range of movement. Consciously differerentiate between the tensing and relaxing of the muscles of the stomach, pelvis and bottom. Deliberately extend your cervical spine by tilting your head slightly.

Tip
■ Try to draw your pelvis into the movement with your lumbar spine. Leave your thoracic spine on the floor at first.

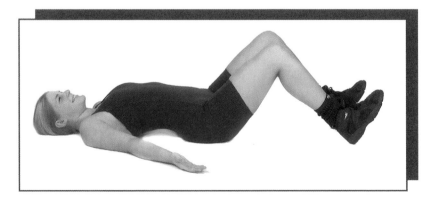

10 Proprioception and spinal posture

TRAINING GOAL **Awareness** of spinal posture
Awareness of individual vertebrae
Flexibility of the spine

Description
Starting position: Take up the "basic all fours position".
Exercise: Round your entire spine and pull your chin into your chest. Then carry out the opposite movement and pull your head back into the nape of your neck.

Tip
▬ Carry out the movements of the spine smoothly and without pressure. Do not push to extremes, but make a harmonious flowing rocking movement with your spine.

Variations
a. Tilt and straighten your pelvis only and then straighten it again.
b. Consciously alternate between tensing and relaxing your stomach, pelvis and buttock muscles.
c. Deliberately breathe in your back or into certain points of your spine.

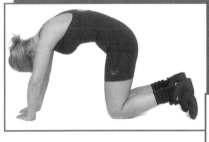
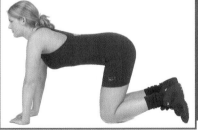

33

11 Proprioception and spinal position

TRAINING GOAL   **Awareness** of spinal position
Awareness of separate vertebrae
Flexibility of the spine

Description
Starting position: Adopt the "Basic Standing" position.
Exercise: Move your pelvis backwards and forwards in isolation. Notice the changes in the whole spine. Press your hands on your pelvic bones when moving your pelvis.

Tips
■■ Bend and straighten your knees in contrast to the forwards and backwards movement of your pelvis. Notice any changes that occur as you do so.

■■ Carry out all the described exercises in the form of "contrast learning" to obtain the correct, physiologically favourable and economical posture. In changing between the two end points of a medium position, acquire a middle position that corresponds to an optimal posture. This contrast will then enable you to find your optimal position and you will be able to discern possible incorrect positions.

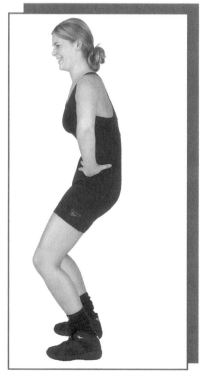

5 The Training Session

The Most Important Exercise Principles

How must an effective training programme be put together?
You want to look after your back. For this, see the listed exercise principles
to improve your fitness and health effectively:
■ Train regularly, at least 2 or 3 times per week!
■ Do not overestimate yourself! Increase the training volume slowly!
■ Vary your training!
■ Carry out the exercises in a controlled way!
■ Adopt the correct starting position!
■ Consider your current state of fitness!

Which exercises are suitable?
Not every exercise is suitable for everyone. To start with, see the section
on stretching and strengthening exercises without equipment. Depending
on your state of fitness and your experience, choose the most relevant
exercises for you.

If you want to increase the level of difficulty, first of all carry out more
repetitions, or hold the adopted position for longer, according to the case.
While carrying out the exercises, gradually supplement your training with
exercises with the bar.

Which advice should be given on breathing?
Do not hold your breath while carrying out the exercises. Try to breathe
deliberately and calmly, even when this might be difficult. Breathe out
during the build-up of tension in the exercise, breathe in when the
exercise is finished and you return to the starting position. As a tip to
avoid stressed breathing, count your breathing rate. This enables you to
regulate the load.

What importance do injuries have for training?
Should you suffer from acute complaints or already have injuries to certain
organs, but nevertheless are interested in training, discuss this with your
doctor beforehand.

When should you stop an exercise?

Stop the exercises at the right time. If you notice that in certain exercises you always have problems in adopting the correct starting position, in bracing or do not carry out the exercise correctly, you should stop exercising immediately. Reread the instructions carefully and learn more about the exercise in the tips provided. If there is no improvement, ask a biomechanist or a physiotherapist for advice.

In any case, you should stop the exercise immediately if you feel any pain.

Tips and requirements for the exercises

Make a few preparations:

■ *Plan your back training during the course of the day!*
If you are interested in training your back in a healthy and lasting way, you must ensure that training is carried out regularly. Ideally, arrange a fixed training time with a partner when you will not be disturbed.

■ *Wear suitable and comfortable clothes!*
Wear real sports clothes for training that are comfortable and in which you can move freely.

■ *Choice of shoes!*
You should always wear shoes for exercising if you are running or hopping. The wearing of shoes is particularly important on wet floors. For stretching and strengthening exercises, shoes are not necessary. For relaxation exercises, on the other hand, you should always take your shoes off.

■ *Setting up the exercise area!*
To be able to carry out an effective exercise programme, make enough room for yourself so that you can lie on the floor and also walk or run a few strides. Move sharp-edged objects or pieces of furniture that can fall over easily away from the exercise area.

■ *Pay attention to the exercise tips!*
Read the extra tips as well as the exercise descriptions.

B TRAINING PROGRAMMES

⊞ Mobility Exercises - Keeping the Main Joints Mobile

Topics
■ Training principles for the development of joint mobility
■ Basic exercises for the improvement of spinal mobility
■ Complementary mobility exercises for the large joints

Focus
Get to know the exercises that improve your joint mobility. Along with the development of spinal mobility, you will also be shown exercises intended to mobilise the legs and shoulders. Our natural movement is always made up of movement chains. In this way, movement restrictions in neighbouring joints directly affect the mobility of the spine. Therefore, in back training, an optimal functional capability of all joints and muscles must also be achieved, so that they can all work better together in daily life.

The described exercises form a programme, but they nevertheless have a complementary nature. For example, in back training they can be used as light relief after strengthening, or as an introduction to training after the warm-up.

Requirements
■ A deliberate exercise execution
■ A sensitive awareness of the body
■ A stable starting position
■ A gentle feeling for the movement potential of the joints

37

1 Training Principles

The exercises to improve mobility of the large joints should always be integrated into your training programme. As well as constituting a self-contained exercise circuit for the development of mobility, these exercises are particularly important to balance strenuous and hard training phases. As well as increasing mobility, they also have an unburdening, relaxing and regenerating effect.

The exercise principles for the development of mobility
Basically it is as vital as when doing stretching exercises that you begin your movement from a fixed point, in order to mobilize optimally and correctly. The moving parts of the body are always anchored when carrying out mobility exercises.

The movements suggested below can for the most part also be combined with each other as variations. However, such combinations often result in the loss of correct mobility due to an accumulation, since the start and finish of the movement come closer together, i.e. they are not the optimal distance from each other during the movement.

Please refer to the following tips regarding the general performance of the exercises.
- Carry out the recommended joint mobilising exercises from a stable and correct starting position.
- Feel the joint mobilisation and trace the movements.
- Carry out the mobilising movements consciously.
- Carry out the exercises slowly, harmoniously and under control. Gradually increase the movement amplitude and reduce it slowly. Jerky and pulling movements are definitely to be avoided.
- Do not look for the extreme point of your mobility. The aim should always be optimal, not maximal mobility.
- Exercise for about 30 seconds on each side of the body. The exercise duration can be increased throughout, according to subjective movement impressions and effects.
- Breathe evenly while you exercise.

■ Notice the movement stimulation in the joints and in the musculature around the joints.

■ Finish the exercise slowly in reverse order.

■ Stop the exercise if you feel pain or if the exercise does not feel correct.

■ In the case of joint injury, clear a possible exercise choice and execution with a movement specialist. Under no circumstances should you adopt a compensating movement for any length of time, where you try to avoid using a joint.

2 Exercises

12 Mobility exercise

TRAINING GOAL   **Mobilising** the Cervical Spine

Description
Starting position: Stand upright with your feet hip-width apart. Stretch your cervical spine upwards.

Exercise: Move your head from left to right, while looking straight ahead.

Tips
- Abide by the individual movement directions of the head.
- Circle your head only in the front semi-circle. Stop circling the head when it reaches the shoulders.
- To start the respective counter-movement, always take your head back to the central position. Do not move it to extremes.

Variation
a. Move your chin towards your chest and centrally backwards and upwards.

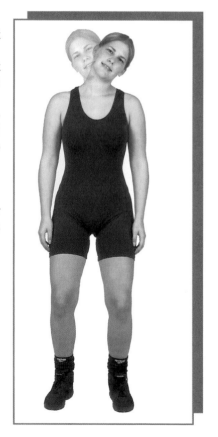

13 Mobility exercise

TRAINING GOAL **Mobilising** the shoulder

Description

Starting position: Stand up straight with your feet hip-width apart. Extend your cervical spine upwards. Place your hands on your shoulders.

Exercise: Slowly circle your arms backwards and upwards and then right forwards and downwards.

Tips

- Carry out the circling movements slowly.
- Aim for a large, controlled range of movement.
- Keep the spine upright.

Variations

a. Move your shoulders diagonally from forwards and upwards to downwards and backwards.
b. Circle your shoulders forwards.
c. Carry out all exercises with straight arms.

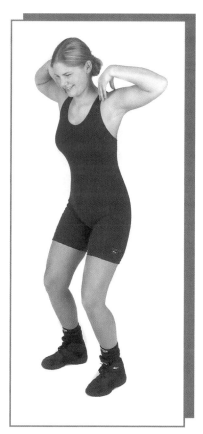

14 Mobility exercise

TRAINING GOAL   **Mobilising** the shoulders
Mobilising the thoracic and cervical spine
Awareness of spinal posture

Description
Starting position: Stand up straight with your feet apart. Stretch your arms out to the sides.
Exercise: Turn your arms alternately forwards and backwards around the longitudinal axis. Your thoracic and cervical spine follow the movement.

Tips
■■ Let your thoracic and cervical spine follow the movement of your shoulder girdle.
■■ Be deliberately aware of the connection between the vertebrae.

Variation
a. Move your shoulder girdle to each side alternately with an erect spine. Keep your legs stable.

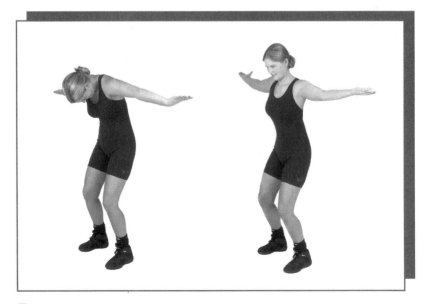

15 Mobility exercise

TRAINING GOAL   **Mobilising** the spine
                 Relaxing the spine

Description
Starting position: From an upright position, bend your spine forwards and downwards.

Exercise: Gradually straighten up vertebra by vertebra until you are standing up straight.

Tips
- Let your trunk hang, loosen your muscles from shoulders, neck, arms with small shaking movements.
- During the rolling-up movement, place your hands on your knees for support.
- Keep your knees bent for a long time. Don't straighten them until you are standing up.
- At the end of the rolling-up movement, circle your shoulders backwards.

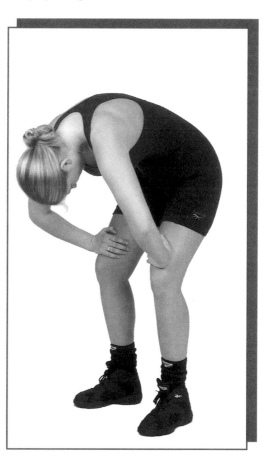

16 Mobility exercise

TRAINING GOAL **Mobilising** the spine

Description
Starting Position: Stand up straight with your feet hip-width apart. Stretch your cervical spine upwards.

Exercise: Turn alternately to each side, keeping your pelvis stable throughout.

Tips
- Only turn your spine, without additionally twisting sideways or forwards.
- Tense your stomach and bottom muscles to stabilise the pelvis.
- Breathe calmly and evenly. Breathe in and out as you turn your torso.

Variation
a. Bend your torso alternately to the sides.

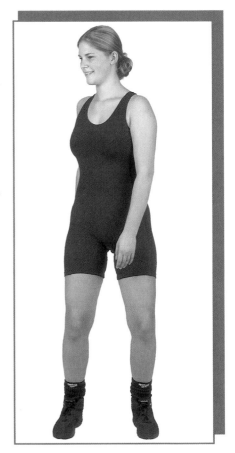

17 Mobility exercise

TRAINING GOAL   **Mobilising** the thoracic spine
Awareness of posture

Description
Starting position: Stand up straight with your feet hip-width apart. Stretch your cervical spine upwards.
Exercise: Move your thoracic spine alternately forwards and upwards and downwards and backwards.
Place your index finger on your sternum to assist the movement. Push your sternum forwards and upwards against the pressure of your finger. In the opposite direction, press your finger downwards and backwards onto your sternum.

Tips
▬▬ Move your cervical and lumbar spine as little as possible, but concentrate hard on the mobility of the thoracic spine.
▬▬ You will find another exercise to mobilise the lumbar spine in the standing position in the following chapter.

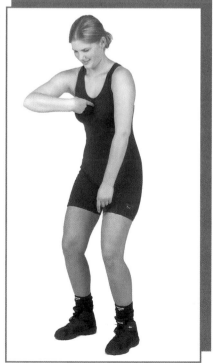

18 Mobility exercises

TRAINING GOAL   **Mobilising** the lumbar spine
Stretching the lateral torso muscles

Description
Starting position: Lie on your back on the floor. Put your legs together and draw them up, keeping your feet on the floor. Your shoulder girdle keeps contact with the floor throughout.
Exercise: Rotate the legs together from left to right.

Tips
■ Your arms lie either in a u-position near the head, or stretched out to the sides near the body. The palms of your hands always face upwards.
■ Your shoulders, elbows and arms remain on the floor. Time the movement of your legs to allow this. To improve your mobility, you must always have a fixed point.
■ Keep your legs close together.
■ Carry out the movement slowly and evenly. Do not stop when changing direction.

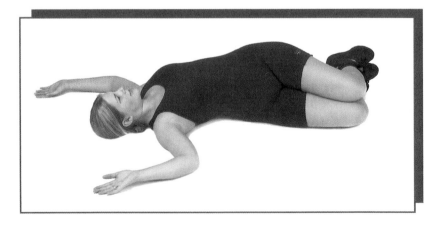

19 Mobility exercise

TRAINING GOAL   **Mobilising** the thoracic spine
                       Stretching the lateral torso muscles

Description

Starting position: Lie on your back on the floor.
                       Pull your bent legs into your chest; raise your feet off the floor.
                       Your shoulders remain on the floor throughout.
Exercise: Rotate your legs together from left to right.

Tips

■ Your arms lie either in the u-position near the head or stretched out to the side near the body. The palms of your hands always face upwards.
■ Your shoulders, elbows and arms remain on the floor. Time the movement of your legs so this is possible.
■ Keep your legs close together.
■ Carry out the movement slowly and evenly.

Variation

a. Reverse the exercise: Keep your legs on the floor to one side and turn your torso and arms to the other side.

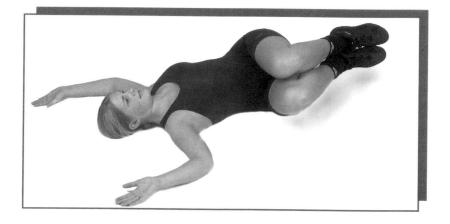

20 Mobility exercises

TRAINING GOAL   **Mobilising** the hips
                   Development of balance

Description
Starting position: Stand up straight with your feet hip-width apart.
Exercise: Circle your bent leg around the hip joint upwards and
                       to the side then downwards again.

Tips
- Keep your pelvis stable, your lumbar spine upright.
- Stare at a fixed point and take outstretched arms out to the side, in order to keep your balance.

Variations
a. Carry out the leg movement forwards and backwards.
b. This movement can also be carried out in the sitting or lying position.

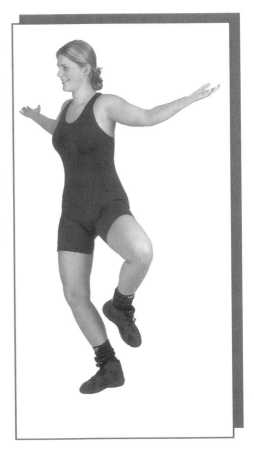

48

21 Mobility exercise

TRAINING GOAL   **Mobilising** the knees and ankles
Developing balance

Description

Starting position: Stand up straight with your feet hip-width apart.
Balance on one leg.

Exercise: Bend and straighten your knee and ankle, imitating a kicking action.
Stretch your arms out to the sides to keep your balance.

Tips

- Keep your pelvis stable, and your lumbar spine straight.
- If necessary, place the tip of your toes on the floor between each kicking movement in order to come back to a stable standing position.

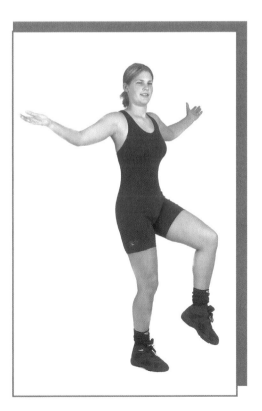

Variations

a. Carry out your leg movement forwards and backwards.
b. Lift the inside and outside of your feet alternately.

49

IV Stretching Exercises – an Important Counter Balance to Muscle Strengthening

Topics
■ The training principles of stretching.
■ The basic exercises to improve the stretchability of the muscles surrounding the spine.
■ The complementary stretching exercises for the large muscle groups.

Emphasis
Familiarise yourself with the different exercises that are necessary for stretching the muscles around the spine. In this way, you will improve your torso and back mobility. In addition, the stretching of the arm, leg, shoulder and hip muscles should be included in your training programme, because the mobility of the muscles and joints surrounding the spine has a direct influence on the posture of your spine. A functionally and physiologically sound deportment and movement of the back can only be assured by an optimal stretchability of the entire muscle system.

To that end, the selection of exercises presented here form a programme in themselves. The training principles of stretching and strengthening go together to correct muscular imbalances. That is why the stretching exercises also represent examples of exercises that can be carried out after strengthening exercises as a balance.

Requirements
■ An appreciation of how to perform each exercise
■ A sensitive feeling for the movement
■ A trusting relationship with the partner in pair-work exercises

1 Training Principles

Exercises to improve the stretchability of the muscles should always be integrated into your training programme. In addition, it is also possible to put together a short stretching programme without carrying out strengthening exercises before or afterwards.

The Exercise Principles of Stretching
There are different ways of approaching muscle stretching. Two methods will be presented here:
a. *static-passive* stretching ("stretching")
b. *tensing-relaxing* stretch (proprioceptive neuromuscular facilitation "PNF method").

Why are both methods described?
Both stretching methods are equally effective. They are both suitable for all target muscles and do not cause injuries. Their difference lies in their position in the exercise programme.

Static-passive stretching is appropriate for warming up or warming down, but in the warm-up programme, an additional integrated muscle warm-up is needed, for example walking or running. Static-passive stretching is especially suitable for beginners, as the gentle movements can be carefully transformed, while developing a sound body awareness by concentrating on the muscles to be stretched.

As well as improving stretchability, PNF stretching also helps to warm up the musculature during the tensing phase preceding stretching. Jogging as a classic way of warming up is not necessary before stretching. According to the sporting activity that follows, it can be carried out afterwards in any case. The main difference between PNF stretching and active-passive stretching is that it consists of three phases, i.e. muscle tensing, a short muscle relaxation and subsequent muscle stretching, which corresponds to the last stretching phase of the static stretching. PNF stretching, equally safe and easy to learn, is consequently more suitable for the advanced who already have a certain experience of exercising. It makes muscles stretching feel easier, as a result of the pre-tensing (due to neuromuscular connections).

How are the stretching methods performed?

a. **static-passive** stretching

■ Warm up thoroughly beforehand with the warm-up programme. Alternatively, you can also warm up by walking or running on the spot, or moving forwards, or by loose and bouncy hops with a soft landing or by dynamic arm swinging in different directions.

■ Ideally, you should stretch twice in each training session: first after warming up to prepare for the ensuing muscular demand in the strengthening phase, and second to end the training session before the relaxation phase.

The first time you stretch, you enable the muscle to lengthen and thereby reach optimal strength during the strengthening phase.

The second stretching phase after muscle strengthening is very important: it enables the previously used musculature to reduce the metabolic waste, so that the muscle can return to its usual length. The second stretching phase can either take place at the end of the whole strengthening phase or after each exercise.

■ Make sure that each stretch is carried out correctly, from the right starting position.

■ Stretch slowly. Avoid jerky movements.

■ Hold the stretch position for 20-30 seconds.

■ Breathe evenly throughout.

■ Be aware of the changing stretch stimulus in the muscles.

■ Finish the stretch slowly in the opposite direction.

■ Always carry out each exercise twice for each side of the body.

■ Talk to your partner during pair work exercises.

■ If you feel pain or discomfort, stop the exercise.

■ Do not stretch injured muscles.

b. *Tensing –relaxing stretching* ("PNF method")

■ This stretching method consists of three phases: tensing, relaxing and stretching.

■ In the tensing phase, the muscle contracts, i.e., you perform the corresponding counter movement to the ensuing stretch position, and notice how the muscle contracts (e.g. the front of the thigh is stretched when the knee bends; to tense it, you must then straighten the knee). The phase lasts about 5-7 seconds.

■ In the relaxation phase, stop tensing and let the muscle rest for about 2-3 seconds.

■ The real stretching then follows, according to the static-passive stretching model, which you can read about above.

2 The Exercises

22 Stretching exercise

TRAINING GOAL   **Stretching** the front and back neck muscles

Description
Starting position: Stand up straight with your feet hip-width apart. Stretch your cervical spine upwards.
Exercise: Move your chin towards your chest.

Tips
■ Control the direction of movement of the head (classic stretch of the front and back of the neck in all four directions).
■ Move your head slightly backwards centrally for the counter movement. Do not aim for extreme end positions; open your mouth if necessary.
■ If you feel uncomfortable during the movement, decrease the range of movement or stop the exercise altogether.

Variation
a. Tilt your head to the side, without twisting it.   To increase the stretch, pull the opposite arm downwards.

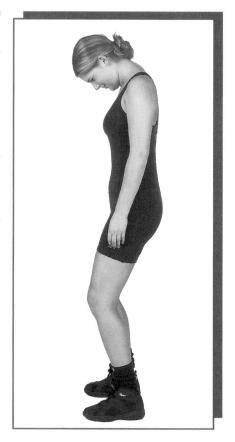

23 Stretching exercise

Training Goal   **Stretching** the front and back neck muscles
                         Relaxation of the muscles of the cervical spine

Description
Starting position: Stand upright with your feet hip-width apart. Your
                         cervical spine is stretched.
                         Place the tips of your fingers behind your ears at the
                         base of your skull.
Exercise: Push the back of your head gently upwards with your
                         fingers, thereby stretching your cervical spine.

Tips

- Turn your knees towards your chest
- Your elbows point right out to the side, your shoulders are simultaneously turned outwards and pulled downwards.
- Relax your neck muscles with small circling and stretching movements after the exercise. You will feel looser.
- **Do not allow** your hands to touch behind your head.

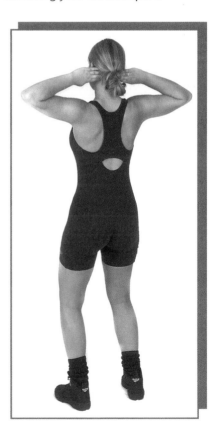

Variation

a. *Tensing-relaxing stretching:*
   Prior to the described stretching exert a slight pressure on your fingers with the back of your head, thereby tensing your front and back neck muscles. You will have a pleasant feeling of relaxation in the following relaxing stretching.

55

24 Stretching exercise

TRAINING GOAL **Stretching** the front and back neck muscles

Description

Starting position: Stand up straight with your feet hip-width apart.
Bend your head to one side, while still looking straight ahead, and place the opposite arm in a slightly rounded position in front of your body.

Exercise: With the other hand, pull your arm forwards and stretch the neck and shoulder muscles.

Tips

- Hold your opposite arm level with your navel and away from the body.
- Your shoulders are both turned outwards and pulled downwards.
- *Point of awareness:*
  In this exercise, the classic neck stretch pulling the head with the hands, is deliberately not used. Pulling the arm reinforces the stretching effect.

Variation

a. Pull your opposite arm diagonally downwards and forwards, level with the pubic bone.

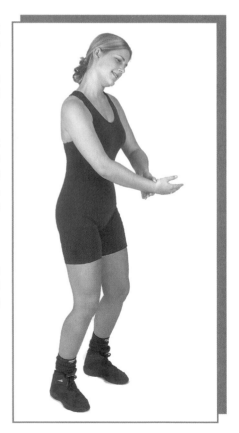

25 Stretching exercise

TRAINING GOAL — **Stretching** the neck and shoulder muscles

Description

Starting position: Stand up straight with your feet hip-width apart. Straighten your neck.
Push your slightly curved right arm forwards and to the side, the palm of the hand upwards.

Exercise: Now turn your head slowly in a narrow arc over your right shoulder.
Key concept "Look scornfully behind you".

Tips

- Pull your chin into your body and keep your face perpendicular.
- Keep your shoulder girdle horizontal; pull your shoulders slightly downwards.

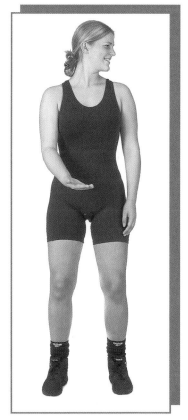

57

26 Stretching exercise

TRAINING GOAL **Stretching** the levator scapulae

Description

Starting position: Stand up straight with your feet hip-width apart.

Exercise: Tilt your head to one side. At the end of the tilting movement, move your head forwards, so that your chin moves towards your chest.

Tips

- ▄ Notice how when you lean your head forwards, the stretch in the lateral neck muscles moves nearer to the neck, thereby reaching the levator scapulae muscles.
- ▄ Move the head sideways and bend it forwards successively.
- ▄ Keep your shoulder girdle horizontal; your shoulders pull slightly downwards.
- ▄ If you carry out the movement correctly, you will feel that the opposite shoulder is pulled slightly upwards. You can also carefully sense the muscle that is being stretched.

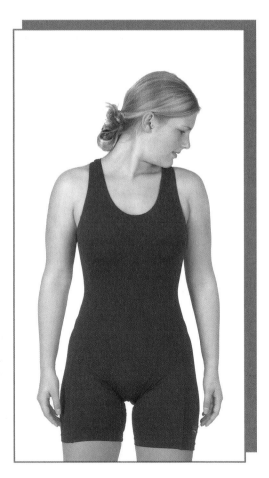

27 Stretching exercise

TRAINING GOAL   **Stretching** the shoulder blade muscles
Stretching the shoulder blade fixators

Description

Starting position: Stand up straight with your feet hip-width apart and your shoulders turned slightly outwards.
Hold your right arm in front of your body at shoulder height, with the forearm in a vertical position.

Exercise: Grip your right upper arm with your left hand and pull the upper arm first forwards, then left to the centre.

Tips

■ Keep the right shoulder in particular turned outwards, pulling it downwards and backwards.

■ *Point of awareness:*
Do not move the right arm to the side, but push it straight forwards.
Your cervical spine remains stretched.

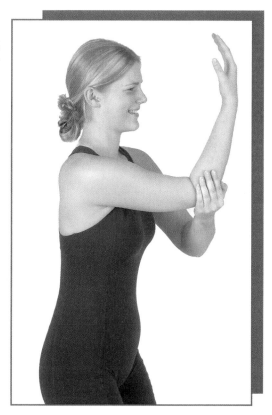

28 Stretching exercise

TRAINING GOAL   **Stretching** the cervical and thoracic spine
Stretching of the shoulder blade fixators

Description
Starting Position: Stand up straight with your feet hip-width apart; your shoulders are turned slightly outwards.
Hold both arms at shoulder height in front of the body, holding your forearms horizontal.
Exercise: Push both elbows right forwards.
Motivation: "Grip a large ball between your arms."

Tips
■ Let your shoulders drop.
■ Keep your cervical spine extended.
■ *Point of awareness:*
If you keep your back straight during this exercise, this strengthens the entire back extension musculature.
■ At the end, relax your shoulders by swinging your arms.

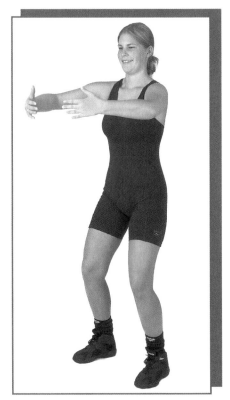

29 Stretching exercise

TRAINING GOAL **Stretching** the chest musculature

Description
Starting position: Place your right foot forwards, in the stride position. Look straight ahead.

Exercise: Bring the right arm horizontally backwards.

Tips
■■ Your shoulder girdle is fixed and remains facing the front.
■■ Your cervical spine is extended.

Variations
a. Flex your wrist inwards and downwards at the end of the arm movement. This will stretch the wrist flexor muscles.
b. Place the rear arm against a wall and turn your shoulder girdle away from the wall.

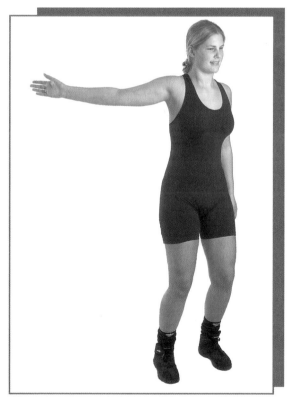

30 Stretching exercises with a partner

TRAINING GOAL   **Stretching** the chest muscles

Exercise: One partner carries out the exercise, the other supports and reinforces.

Description
Starting position: Sit up straight on the floor and place your arms in a u-shape above your head.
                       Your partner places the outside of one leg against your back, thus supporting your upright sitting posture.
Exercise: Your partner slowly moves your arms backwards at shoulder height.

Tips
■ Hold the palms of your hands perpendicular, with your thumbs pointing backwards.
■ Extend your cervical spine.
■ Your partner moves your arms backwards only. Do not push your shoulders upwards.
■ Your partner ensures that his own back posture is correct (bent over with straight back!).

Variations
Before stretching, you can perform the following movements according to the PNF stretching method:
a. Try to bring your arms inwards and forwards from the u-position. Your partner resists this, and there is a balance of strength.
b. Relax your arms. Your partner grips your upper arms or your wrists and starts to relax your arms with light, tiny, but fast shaking movements.

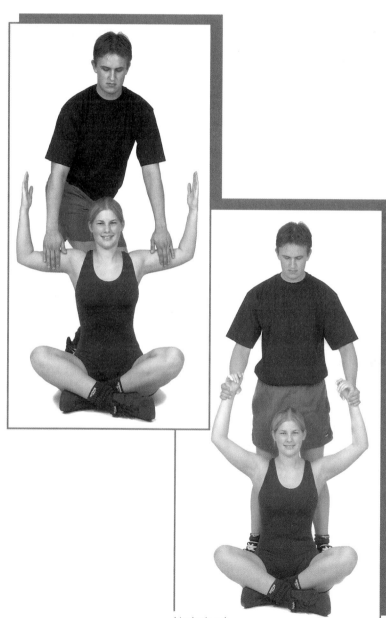

Variation b.

31 Stretching exercise

TRAINING GOAL **Stretching** the arm extensor muscles

Description
Starting position: Stand comfortably with your spine erect.
Exercise execution: Massage the connection of the shoulder muscle and the arm extensor muscle (triceps).

Tips
- This kind of muscles relaxation of the upper arm is often sufficient. Besides, it is much more important to strengthen the arm extensor muscle (triceps) than to stretch it, as it is more inclined to be weak than the antagonist, more easily shortenened arm flexor muscle (biceps).
- *Important remark:* Stretching is only useful after heavy loading of the arm extensor muscle (for example by strengthening exercises with an exercise band), as the cervical spine will be simultaneously increasingly loaded by overstretching it. (see variation a).

Variation
a. In an upright posture, with the cervical spine extended, bend one arm and take it behind the head. With the other hand, grip the elbow of that arm and pull it slowly past the back of the head.

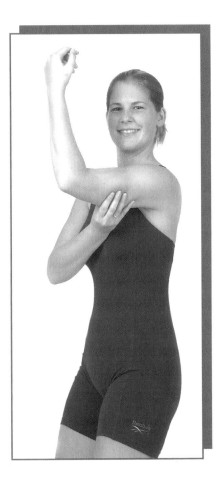

32 Stretching exercise

TRAINING GOAL   **Stretching** the wrist flexor muscles

Description
Starting position: Stand up straight with the feet hip-width apart.
Bring your right arm forwards and tip your wrist downwards.
Exercise: Grasp the palm and fingers of your right hand with your left hand.
Slowly stretch your right arm against the resistance of the left.

Tips
- Also grasp your thumbs.
- You can also comfortably carry out this exercise in an upright sitting position.
- **Important Remark:** This exercise prepares the wrist muscles well for the starting position "on all fours" (see exercise 5).

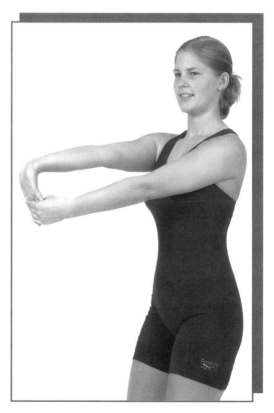

33 Stretching exercise

TRAINING GOAL   **Stretching** the lateral torso muscles
                   Stretching the wide back muscles (latissimus dorsi)

Description
Starting position: Stand up straight with your feet hip-width apart and your legs slightly bent, your hips are tilted.
                       Stretch one arm upwards.
Exercise: **Classic torso muscle stretch:** Incline your upper body to the side, while keeping your pelvis stable. Your arm aims for the diagonal.

Tips
■ Tense your stomach and buttock muscles, so that they remain in the lateral plane of movement and do not deviate forwards or backwards.
■ *Point of awareness:* Try to move your arm higher and higher, not only to the side. Your elbows push further and further diagonally.
   Do not rest your lower hand on your pelvic ridge, but bring your arm past your body, with the palm of the hand upwards (turn the shoulder outwards).
■ "Undo" the stretch in reverse order.

Variations
After the classic form described, there are two other possibilities which are simultaneously associated with an intensive strengthening of the opposite torso muscle chain (long spinal erectors, latissimus dorsi muscles, lumbar muscles, oblique abdominal muscles):
a. In a standing position, place both arms above the head shoulder-width apart. Bend to the left, while pushing your right arm diagonally.
    Now press your left arm against an imaginary heavy mass towards your left knee and then press against, a heavy iron ball diagonally in a distant circle, again from above hip-height upwards. Repeat this movement with the left arm up to ten times.

b. As variation a., now use real weights during the exercise, for example a dumbbell or a wrist weight.

c. Stand up straight and grip your right wrist with your left hand above your head. Tense your stomach and lower torso muscles. Now pull your right arm to the left side, to a horizontal position. Intensify the stretch, so that your right elbow pushes even further diagonally.

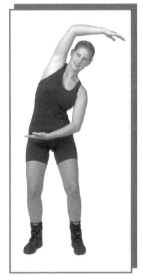

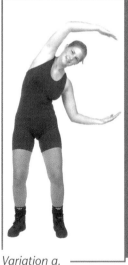

Variation a.

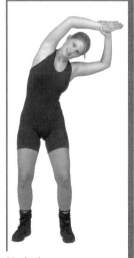

Variation c.

34 Stretching exercise

TRAINING GOAL   **Stretching** the back muscles
Stretching the quadratus lumborum
Stretching the lumbar spine

Description
Starting position: Sit on your heels and extend your arms far forwards, body-width apart.
Your bottom remains on your calves, pull your chin towards your chest and extend your cervical spine upwards.
Exercise: Press (simultaneously or alternately) your hands hard onto the floor and then crawl little by little, centimetre by centimetre forwards with your fingertips.

Tips
■ Keep your bodyweight deliberately backwards and downwards, thus keeping your lumbar spine stable.
■ The stretch on the spine is only gradually perceptible. Be very patient.
■ The exercise can take up to 2 minutes per side.

Variations
a. **Additional exercise:** turn your hands outwards, so that the palms of your hand stay perpendicular and the thumbs point to the floor. Keep your hand far forwards and drop your elbows slowly to the floor without pressure.
   This stretches the inner shoulder muscles as well as the chest muscles
b. As variation a., but now push your elbows out to the side with your hands.

Ineffective exercise
■ Avoid the classic "back rocking" stretch, as it overextends and overloads the lumbar spine.

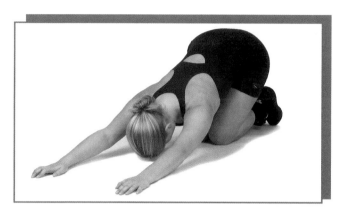

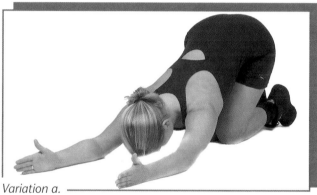

Variation a.

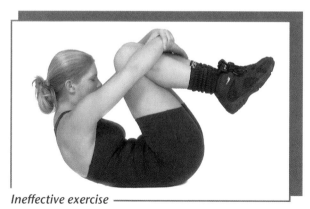

Ineffective exercise

69

35 Stretching exercise

TRAINING GOAL   **Stretching** the lateral back muscles
Stretching the quadratus lumborum
Extension of the lumbar spine

Description
Starting position: Sit on your heels and stretch your arms forwards, body-width apart.
Your bottom remains right on your calves, pull your chin into your chest. Stretch your cervical spine.
Exercise: "Walk" your hands from a central position far to the left. Now place your bottom on the opposite calf, pushing down on the right heel, while your hands remain on the floor.

Tips
■ Take your time over this exercise. Notice how much tension disappears from your back and particularly from your lumbar spine.
■ This exercise also works by reducing the arm mobility in the shoulder joint.

Variations
a. As described, but now press the right hand on the floor and let the left elbow (and with it the whole forearm) drop loosely to the floor, slightly bent, without relaxing the hand.
b. As described, but now also push the right elbow outwards, while letting the left elbow drop back to the floor.
c. *PNF stretch with additional strengthening:* Lift your left arm straight slightly off the floor, so that the palm of your hand remains perpendicular and the thumbs point to the ceiling. Meanwhile, push your right hand hard against the floor.
Hold this position for a while - up to 10 seconds - before returning to the described stretch.

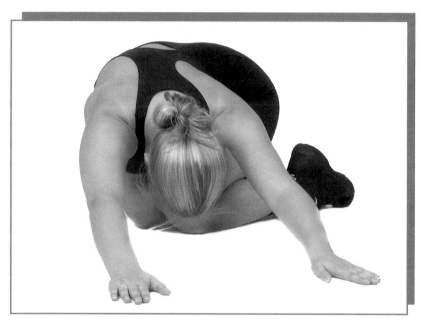

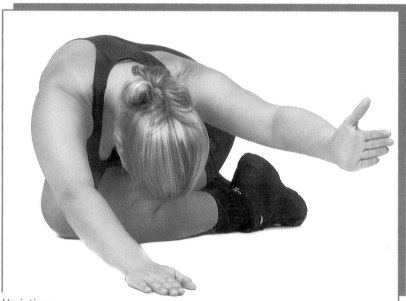

Variation c.

36 Stretching exercise with a partner

TRAINING GOAL   **Stretching** the quadratus lumborum
Extension of the lumbar spine

Exercise Situation: One partner carries out the exercise; the other assists the stretch.

Description
Starting position: Lie relaxed on your back on the floor.
Your partner bends over with a straight back and places your lower legs on his thighs and presses them firmly into his waist with his elbows.
Exercise: With a slight transfer of weight, your partner pulls hard on your legs, pelvis and your lumbar spine.

Tips
■ Gently resist your partner's pull with your hands on the floor. Lie on a mat.
■ Your bottom can be slightly raised from the floor. But even without raising your bottom from the floor, your lumbar spine will be stretched passively.
■ Do not help actively. The stretch happens only when your partner pulls your legs.

Variation
a. At the beginning and throughout, your partner can relax your muscles through small shaking movements.

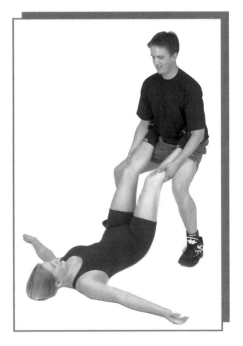

37 Stretching exercise

TRAINING GOAL	**Stretching** the chest muscles
	Stretching the oblique abdominal muscles
	Mobility of the spine

Description

Starting position: Lie on your side on the floor.
Bend your bottom leg at right angles at the knee and hip; straighten the top leg in line with the body.

Exercise: Turn the bottom shoulder and arm backwards and lay down both arms bent at the elbows.
Lay the head likewise turned backwards on the floor.

Tips

■ Hold this position for 1-2 minutes (twisting stretch on stomach).
■ Keep your top leg on the floor.
■ If necessary, place a flat cushion under your head.

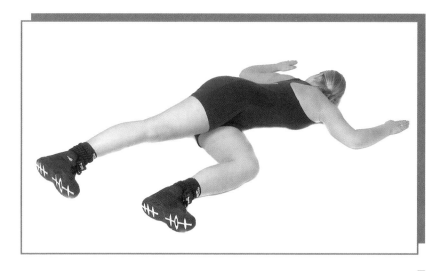

73

38 Stretching exercise

TRAINING GOAL   **Stretching** the chest muscles
Stretching the oblique abdominal muscles
Mobility of the spine

Description
Starting position: Lie on your side with your legs bent on the floor. Your arms are also bent and lie one on top of the other.
Exercise: Turn the top shoulder slowly backwards, bringing with it the top bent arm, until it gradually drops to the floor.
Your head follows the movement.

Tips
■ Start with your arms on the floor bent in the u-position.
■ *Point of awareness:* Both knees must always be kept firmly on the floor when you turn back.
■ If your arm position is comfortable, then lay your arm straight behind your head.
■ Hold this position for a while; let the whole arm, including the shoulder, drop slowly down to the floor under the effect of gravity.

Variations
There are further ways of intensifying the stretch by varying the starting position:
a. Start by lying on your side and stretch out your bottom leg in line with the body and place the top knee bent firmly on the floor. In addition, hold your knees with the opposite hand on the floor. Carry out the exercise by turning back your shoulder, arm and head, as described.
b. Start by lying on your side, and lay the top knee on the floor, gripping the thigh of your bottom leg. Carry out the exercise as described.
Lay your arms straight out to the side.

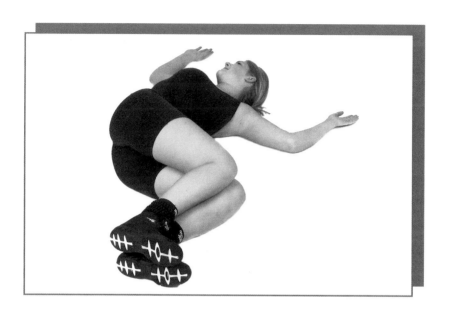

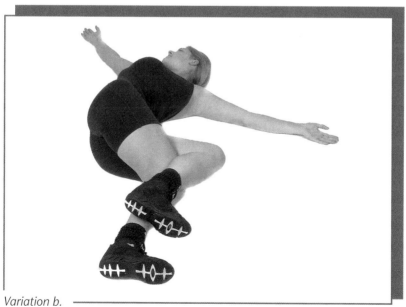

Variation b.

39 Stretching exercise with a partner

TRAINING GOAL   **Stretching** the chest muscles
Stretching the oblique abdominal muscles
Mobility of the spine

Exercise situation: One partner carries out the exercise, the other assists.

Description
Starting position: Lie on your back on the floor and bend your left leg and place it on the floor to the right of your body. Your arms lie on the right side of your body.
Your partner holds your left knee against the floor and grasps your left forearm.
Exercise: Your partner brings your left arm, almost straight over to your left side towards the floor.

Tips
■ Your partner carries out the exercise slowly. The exercise can last up to one minute each side.
■ With the help of your partner, keep your left knee on the floor as a fixed point.

Variations
a. **PNF stretch:** Before your partner moves your arm against the floor, in the starting position, press lightly against his hands with your left arm.
b. Before or during the exercise: lie on your back (also possible on your side). Your partner grasps your left wrist with his hand; with the other hand he supports your elbows. Your partner pulls your arm slightly, and starts to make small, fast shaking movements. Finally, carry out the stretch as described.
c. The stretch is easier if you keep both legs bent on top of each other on the right side (see preceding exercise).

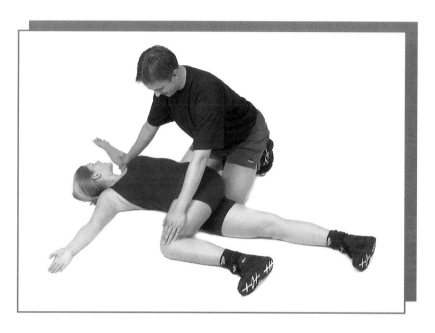

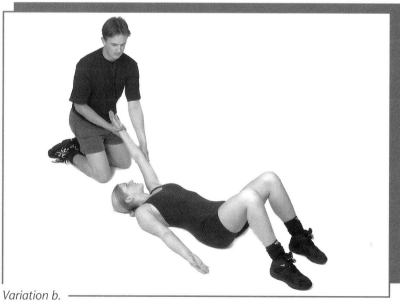

Variation b.

40 Stretching exercise

TRAINING GOAL   **Stretching** the hip flexor muscles

Description

Starting position: Stand in a stride position, your right leg to the rear, your right heel is raised off the floor. Tilt your pelvis strongly, so that the lumbar spine is rounded.

Exercise: Strengthen the described position. Also, you can bend your upper body slightly to the left.

Tips

■ When tilting your pelvis, bring your pelvis backwards with your hands placed on your hips.
■ The hip flexor muscles consist of two parts. With the described exercise, it is above all the part originating from the lumbar spine that is stretched. In the following variation, the part coming from the pelvis bone is stretched.

Variations

a. From a kneeling position, push your bodyweight forwards, with your front foot and back knee far apart. Your upper body is straight; the lumbar spine is flat, then slightly rounded backwards.
b. As described in variation a., you increase the stretch by gripping your rear ankle with your hand and pull your foot towards your bottom. You should place a soft cushion under your rear knee.

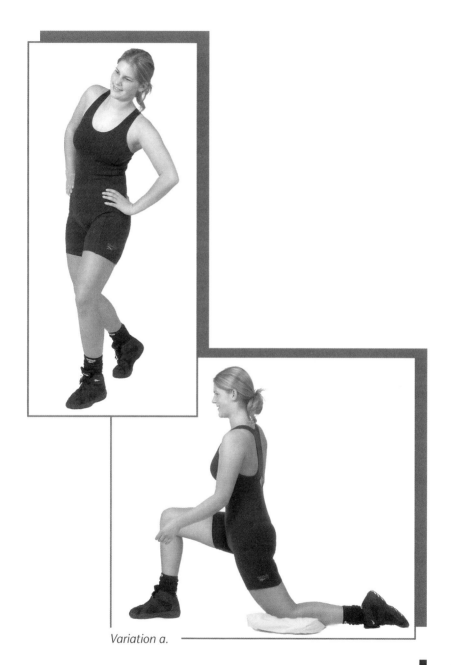

Variation a.

41 Stretching exercise

TRAINING GOAL   **Stretching** the quadriceps muscles

Description

Starting position: Lie on your side on the floor.
                       Your bottom leg is slightly bent; your hips are kept
                       perpendicularly stable and your torso is firm.

Exercise: Grip your top ankle with your hand.
                       Move your foot slowly towards your bottom.

Tips

■ *Point of awareness:* Your lumbar spine is flat or slightly rounded, tense
your torso muscles and clench your buttocks.

■ Do not hollow your back.

Variation

Exercise situation: one partner carries out the exercise, the other assists.

a. Lie on your stomach on the floor. Your partner kneels next to you. He
stabilises with his left hand the contact of your pelvis with the floor,
with the right hand he grips your lower leg.

Your partner moves your lower leg against your thigh, your heels move
towards your bottom.

In case you have knee problems, you and your partner must be very
careful with this exercise. Increase the stretch slowly and do not push
to extremes.

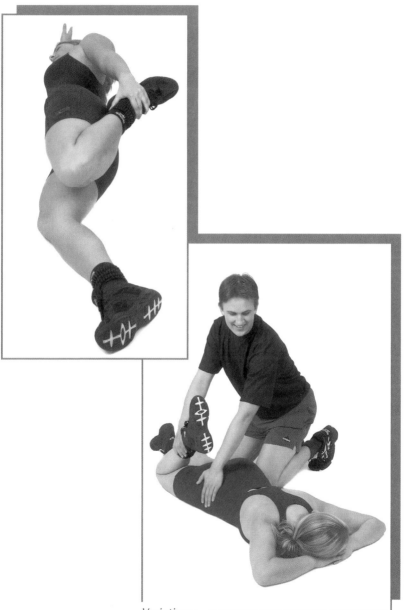

Variation a.

81

42 Stretching exercise

TRAINING GOAL   **Stretching** the inner thigh muscles

Description

Starting position: Lie on your back on the floor.
Lift your legs and hold them at right angles to the floor.

Exercise: Grip your inner thighs with your hands and slowly move your legs downwards and outwards.

Tips

■■ Let gravity work on your knees, as it gradually moves them to the floor.
■■ Your head is relaxed and remains on the floor.
■■ This exercise stretches the short sections of the inner thigh in particular. To stretch the long, two-headed sections of the inner thigh, do variations a. or b. of the exercise.

Variations

a. Sit on the floor and support yourself with your hands behind your back and straighten your spine. Spread your legs and bend your feet, so that your toes are pointing upwards.
Now move your upper body slowly forwards, with an erect spine, and place your hands behind you. Only when you can sit upright, without supporting yourself with your hands, should you lean your upper body centrally forwards towards your legs.

b. Lie on your back on the floor, with your bottom as near as possible to a wall. Now let your legs fall out to the sides against the wall.

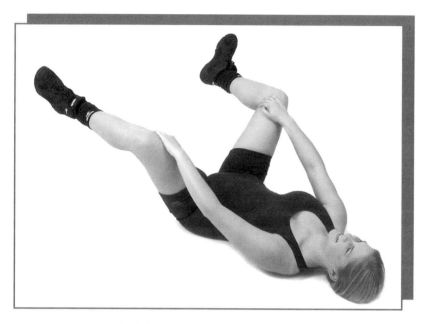

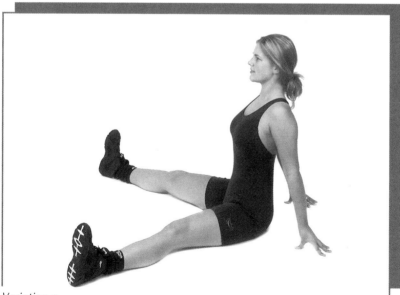

Variation a.

43 Stretching exercise

TRAINING GOAL   **Stretching** the hamstring muscles

Description
Starting position: From a standing position, place one leg in front of you, heel to the ground.
Support yourself with your hands on your other bent leg.
Exercise: Slowly move your erect upper body forwards over the straight leg.

Tips
- *Point of awareness:* Place your hands on your leg with the thumbs pointing downwards, while turning your shoulders outwards and keeping your spine extended.
- Twist the foot of the straight leg slightly inwards and also slightly outwards. Feel how the stretch in the muscle changes. You are aiming for different muscle groups.
- Push your bottom backwards to the right. Stretch with the idea of moving your navel forwards and downwards and stretching the muscle above the bottom.

Variations
Exercise situation: one partner carries out the exercise, the other assists.
a. Lie on your back on the floor. Your partner grips your straight left leg around the calf and the thigh. Your partner brings your straight leg against his upper body. You still lie passive and relaxed on the floor. Your partner feels the resistance to the stretch in your thigh and adapts the pull on your leg accordingly.
b. As described in variation a., you can both bend and stretch your toes.

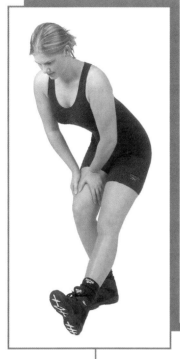

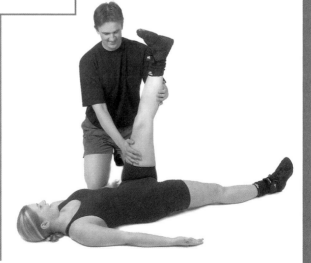

Variation a.

44 Stretching exercise

TRAINING GOAL | **Stretching** the gluteus maximus

Description

Starting position: Lie on your back and cross your legs, so that your right ankle is lying on your left knee.

Exercise: Grip the back of the thigh of the bottom leg with your hands and pull it towards your upper body.

Tips

■ Keep your head and your shoulders relaxed on the floor.

Variation

a. When you push your right knee carefully outwards, the stretch in the right buttock feels even stronger.

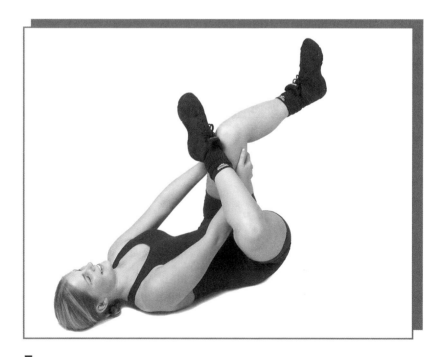

V Strength Training of the Whole Body without Equipment

Topics
▪ Exercise principles of strengthening exercises
▪ Basic exercises to improve muscle strength
▪ Essential starting positions and exercise situations
▪ Effective exercises for vital back and torso stability
▪ Varied pair-work exercises

Focus
Learn the exercises to do alone and in pairs that serve to strengthen weakened muscles and muscle groups. You need no extra equipment to carry out these exercises, i.e. you can do them anywhere. When doing the exercises, note that in this chapter basic principles are presented for the starting positions and how to do the exercises, which you will also see in the next section.

Requirements
▪ Active and upright posture
▪ Correct starting position for the exercises
▪ Intensive warm-up and stretching of the muscles
▪ Appropriate choice of partner for pair- work exercises

1 Training Principles

When are muscles strengthened? – Why should muscles be strengthened?
Muscle strengthening is the key component of any training programme. It often occurs in daily, repetitive actions such as stair climbing or cycling. In order to carry out sporting movements optimally and successfully, a certain degree of muscle strength is also necessary, which can be improved either by the movement itself or by additional, targeted strength training. In the area of general exercise, strengthening exercises are usually carried out to re-strengthen muscles that have been weakened by defective movements in daily life and are not able to carry out their function of protecting and supporting the body. The back and trunk muscles in particular are inclined to be weak due to lack of use. The spine thus lacks the crucial protective function that reduces or protects against damaging loads. An effective exercise programme for the maintenance and improvement of back and torso strength has a remedial and preventive effect.

What is the difference between static and dynamic strengthening?
In contrast to stretching, which is carried out with little movement, in strength training there are two equally correct ways of execution, dependant on the function of the muscles.

One way is to hold the muscles in the strengthening position for a long time. This type should be chosen for muscles that perform mainly supporting work in daily life. This includes the torso muscles in particular. They stabilize an erect and active body posture.

The other way is to carry out exercises dynamically, that means; the muscle length is changed constantly. Dynamic strengthening should be used for the muscles of the limbs, which as a rule perform active work in daily life.

Which training methods should be chosen?
For fitness and health-oriented sport, there are two fundamentally different training methods: muscle building training and strength endurance training.

Muscle building training is defined by high intensity training with few repetitions and many sets. You need additional equipment for training, such as dumbbells, a training band or a training partner, to provide resistance. Usually, 8-10 repetitions of the exercise are performed, all with correct form, in about 5 sets. Muscle building training takes place at the start of a training process.

In strength endurance training, the aim is to prepare the muscles to perform their intended function for as long as possible, and to delay fatigue as long as possible. The training intensity is obviously lower than in muscle building training. The number of repetitions per set is higher, however, at about 12-15 repetitions (that corresponds to around 60% of the maximum number of repetitions with a correct technique). Up to three sets are carried out.

The exercise principles of strength training

- Take care to carry out the exercise correctly.
- Use the static or dynamic method, according to the muscle function.
- A series of static strength training has the following characteristics: hold the position for around 8-15 seconds. Then rest for the same length of time. Now repeat the exercise 5-8 times, according to your state of fitness. Carry out 2 to 3 series per exercise.
- You can also determine the duration of holding by choosing how you breathe. The benefit is that you then consciously breathe in and out continuously.
- One series of dynamic strengthening includes 12-15 repetitions per body side. Perform 3-5 series per exercise. Between series, take a 30-45 second rest.
- Be aware of your body while strengthening.
- Breathe regularly. Avoid any kind of forced breathing. Always strengthen both side of the body. Vary the exercises regularly, so that other muscles are also strengthened.
- Stretch the muscles after strengthening.

2 Exercises for the Back Muscles

45 Strengthening exercise without equipment

TRAINING GOAL   **Strengthening** the back muscles
Awareness of the spine

Description
Starting position: Your legs are straight and the palms of your hands face upwards.
Exercise: Flex your feet and press your legs down onto the floor, also the backs of your hands, arms, and shoulders. Pull your back deliberately towards the floor.

Tips
■ Pull your chin in towards your chest and press the back of your head into the floor.
■ This exercise is especially suitable to be done between intensive strengthening exercises for the abdominal muscles.

Variations
a. Tense your whole body. Raise your bottom, thighs and lumbar spine from the floor.
b. Clench a gymnastic ball between your knees during the exercise.

difficulty
light
medium
hard

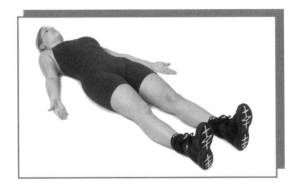

46 Strengthening exercise without equipment

TRAINING GOAL **Strengthening** of the back extensor muscles
Strengthening of the lumbar spine – hip area

Description
Starting position: Take up the "basic prone position".
Exercise: Raise your arms from the floor and bend your wrists back and push your hands down to the floor.

Tips
- Your cervical spine is straight. Look straight down at the floor.
- Raise your upper body as far as the sternum from the floor and keep it raised.
- Move your shoulder blades together and pull them downwards.
- Your feet are flexed and your legs are straight.

Variation
a. Straighten each arm and alternately bring each forwards aligned with the side of the body.

difficulty
light
medium
hard

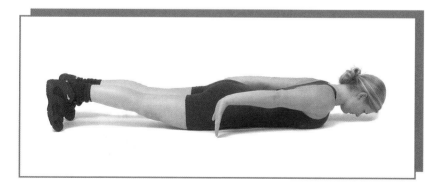

47 Strengthening exercise without equipment

TRAINING GOAL
Strengthening the back extensor muscles
Strengthening the lumbar spine – hip area

Description
Starting position: Take up the "basic prone position".
Your arms are bent in the u-position by your sides.
Exercise: Raise your arms from the floor.

Tips
■ Hold the palms of your hands perpendicular, your thumbs pointing upwards.
■ Your lumbar spine is straight, i.e. more flat than hollow.
■ Your shoulder blades move together and pull downwards.
■ Your feet are flexed, your legs straight.

Variations
a. Push your arms straight forwards in alternation.
b. Raise your straightened legs from the floor in alternation, keeping the heels pushed backwards.
c. Carry out very small but fast upwards and downwards movements with your arms, as if you wanted to chop something small. Keep your torso stable, particularly in the lumbar spine-pelvis-hip area.
d. As described, in addition look under each armpit to the side. During the slight rotation movement in the cervical and thoracic spine area, keep your pelvis stable.
e. As described in variation d, in addition, raise both legs from the floor.

difficulty
light
medium
hard

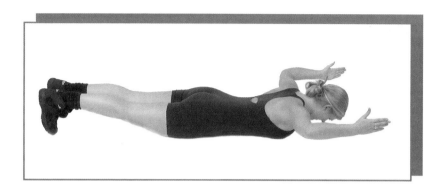

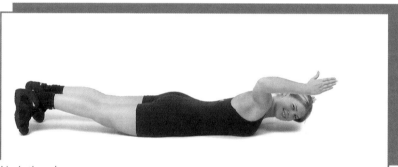

Variation d.

93

48 Strengthening exercises without equipment

TRAINING GOAL   **Strengthening** the back extensor muscles
Strengthening the lumbar – hip area
Strengthening the gluteus maximus

Description

Starting position: Take up the "basic prone position".
Your arms are in the u-position near the body.

Exercise: Straighten your upper body and raise your arms from the floor. Push them alternately straight forwards. At the same time, raise the opposite leg from the floor.

Tips

■ Carry out the changes in the exercise rhythmically.
■ Hold the palms of your hands perpendicularly, your thumbs pointing upwards.
■ Your lumbar spine is straight, i.e. more flat than hollow.

difficulty

easy
medium
hard

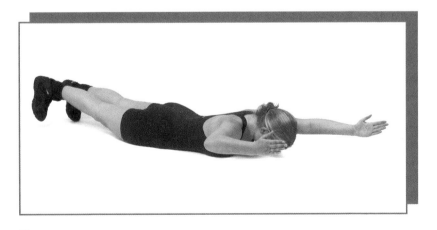

49 Strengthening exercises without equipment

TRAINING GOAL   **Strengthening** the back extensor muscles
Strengthening the lumbar spine - hip area
Strengthening the gluteus maximus

Description

Starting position: Take up the "basic prone position".
Stretch your arms past your head.

Exercise: Raise your arms and legs from the floor.
Open and close your arms and legs simultaneously.

Tips

▪ Keep your arms and legs straight. The palms of your hands are perpendicular; your feet are pulled in.
▪ Your lumbar spine is straight, i.e. it is more flat than hollow. Try to raise your navel slightly from the floor.
▪ Your neck is straight.

Variation

a. Change the rhythm of the leg and arm movements.

difficulty

easy
medium
hard

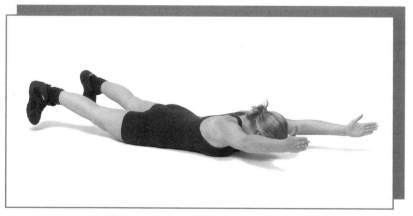

50 Strengthening exercise without equipment

TRAINING GOAL   **Strengthening** the back extensor muscles
Strengthening the shoulder blade muscles
Strengthening the hamstring muscles

Description

Starting position: Take up the "basic kneeling position".
Place the backs of your hands against your bottom.

Exercise: Bend your upper body slowly forwards. At the same time, your bottom moves towards your heels.
Press your hands hard against your bottom.

Tips

■ Pay attention to your balance. Do not squeeze your feet onto the floor for outside support.

■ *Point of awareness*: Keep your back completely straight and stable. While bending forwards, move only the hips, not your lumbar spine.

■ This exercise makes you focus on keeping a straight back while leaning forwards.

Variations

a. As described, but place your hands behind your head, your elbows point right out to the sides. By raising your shoulders as well, you increase the muscle strengthening intensity.

b. As in variation a., now stretch alternately one arm diagonally forwards and upwards. Tilt your perpendicular hand slightly outwards.

difficulty
easy
medium
hard

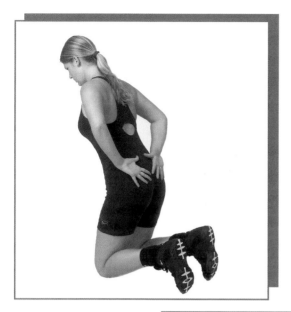

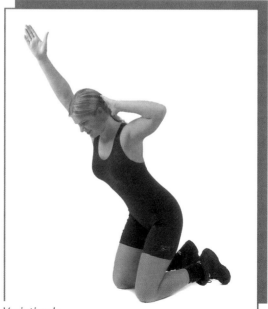

Variation b.

51 Strengthening exercise without equipment

TRAINING GOAL   **Strengthening** the back extensor muscles
Strengthening the shoulder blade muscles

Description
Starting position: Change from the "basic kneeling position" to a one-kneed position.
Increase the distance between your legs.
Exercise: Bend your upper body diagonally forwards, and at the same time push your wrists downwards and forwards, tilting them diagonally downwards and backwards.

Tips
■■ Keep your upper body stable.
■■ Tense your stomach, and avoid overstretching the spine by hollowing your back.

Variation
a. Push your arms forwards and upwards alternately.   Tip your perpendicular wrists slightly outwards.

difficulty
easy
medium
hard

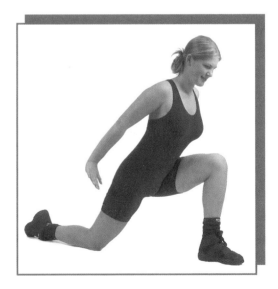

52 Strengthening exercise without equipment

TRAINING GOAL   **Strengthening** the back muscles
Strengthening the gluteus maximus
Strengthening the hamstrings

Description
Starting position: Take up the "basic all fours position". Extend one leg backwards horizontally to the floor and bend your knee at a right angle.
Exercise: Raise and lower your leg, while making small, fast movements with your lower leg.

Tips
▄▄ Keep your back and pelvis stable; do not let your pelvis sag.
▄▄ Flex your foot.

Variation
a. Bend and stretch your knee while keeping your thigh horizontal.

difficulty
easy
medium
hard

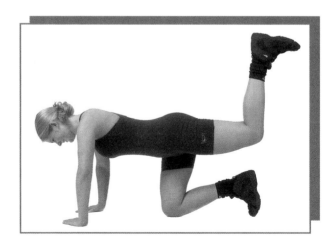

53 Strengthening exercise without equipment

Training Goal   **Strengthening** the back muscles
                        Strengthening the gluteus maximus
                        Strengthening the hamstrings

Description
Starting position: Take up the "basic all fours position".
Exercise: Extend one arm forwards and the opposite leg
                        backwards horizontally to the floor. Hold this position.
                        Bend your arm and leg and bring them together
                        beneath your body.

Tips
■ Your back, including your cervical spine, should be rounded in the bent position.
■ Your arm and your leg must not touch each other beneath your body.
■ In the extended position, flex your foot and keep your hand perpendicular with the thumb upwards and tilted slightly outwards.
■ Keep your back stable in the physiologically most comfortable position.
■ If you have wrist problems in the all fours position, stretch your wrist muscles beforehand.

Variations
a. Stretch and bend your arm or leg only.
b. Hold the extended position and make small, fast movements with your arm and leg, as if you wanted to chop something.

difficulty
easy
medium
hard

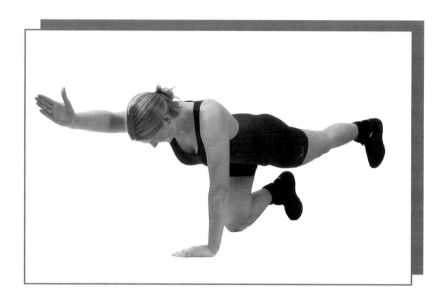

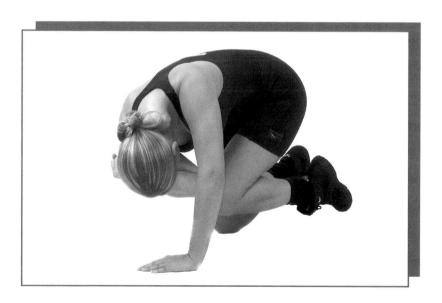

54 Strengthening exercise without equipment

TRAINING GOAL   **Strengthening** the back muscles

Description

Starting position: Sit upright on a stool.
Spread your fingers and place the palm of your hand on your stomach and the back of your hand on your lumbar spine.

Exercise: Bend your upper body forwards. Hold this position for some time. Feel the stability of your upper body with your hands.

Tips

- Keep your back actively straight. Bend only from the hips.
- Your cervical spine is extended in line with the spine.

Variation

a. To intensify the strengthening exercise, carry out different movements with the arms when leaning forwards.

difficulty

easy
medium
hard

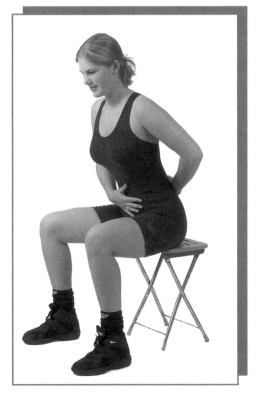

55 Strengthening exercise without equipment

TRAINING GOAL   **Strengthening** the back muscles
Strengthening the latissimus dorsi

Description
Starting position: Take up the "basic straight-backed bent-over position".
Exercise: Swing your bent arms backwards alternately.

Tips
- Hold the rear arm position for a few seconds.
- Keep your back stable.
- Move your arms clearly backwards, so that your shoulder blades move towards your spine.

Variation
a. Swing both arms backwards at the same time.

difficulty
easy
medium
hard

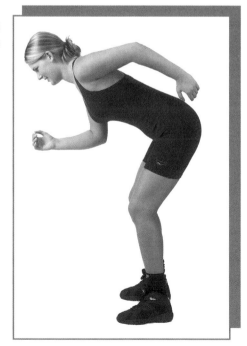

56 Strengthening exercise without equipment

TRAINING GOAL   **Strengthening** the back extensor muscles
                       Strengthening the shoulder blade muscles

Description
Starting position: Take up the "basic straight-backed bent-over
                       position".
                       Push your arms backwards with your hands bent
                       forwards at the wrists.
Exercise: Swing your arms alternately forwards and upwards.
                       Your wrist is now extended and quite perpendicular,
                       your thumb points backwards.

Tips
- Keep your back stable.
- Carry out the arm movement slowly and under control. Hold the final
  positions for a few seconds.
- Tense your abdominal muscles to stop your back from hollowing.
- It is also possible to start the exercise with the feet in the stride
  position, thus improving trunk stability in the lumbar spine-pelvis-hips
  area.

Variations
a. Swing both arms forwards and upwards at the same time.
b. When your upper body is leaning forwards, raise both arms in the u-
   position, hold the palms of your hands together and move your elbows
   clearly backwards.
c. With the upper body, carry out small up and down movements from
   the hips.

difficulty
easy
medium
hard

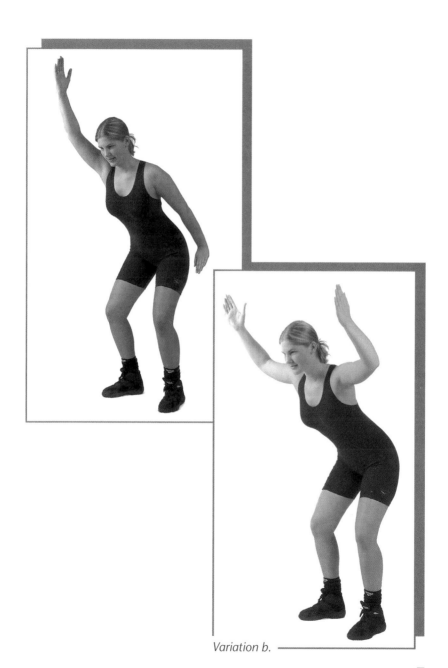

Variation b.

3   Exercises for the Shoulder Muscles

57 Strengthening exercise without equipment

TRAINING GOAL   **Strengthening** the shoulder girdle muscles
                     Strengthening the back muscles

Description
Starting position: Stand up straight with your feet hip-width apart.
                        Bend your arms and hold them in front of your body.
                        Your thumbs point upwards.
Exercise: Pull your elbows backwards on imaginary threads.

Tips
- The tension between your shoulder blades increases. Your shoulder blades move together and pull downwards at the same time.
- *Point of awareness:* tense your lower torso muscles in the stomach and buttocks and keep your spine stable.
- Keep your cervical spine extended upwards.
- Keep your legs slightly bent.

Variations
a. Push your hands and lower arms slowly forwards under tension.
b. Place your hands in the u-position; the palms of your hands face each other. From this position, force your elbows backwards.
c. As described in variation b., hold an exercise band under slight tension between your hands. Force your arms backwards.
d. As described in variation c., bend and stretch your arms at the elbow joint out to the sides and back into the u-position.
e. As described in variation b, bring your arms from the u-position perpendicularly upwards and pull them under tension slowly back downwards into the u-position.

difficulty
easy
medium
hard

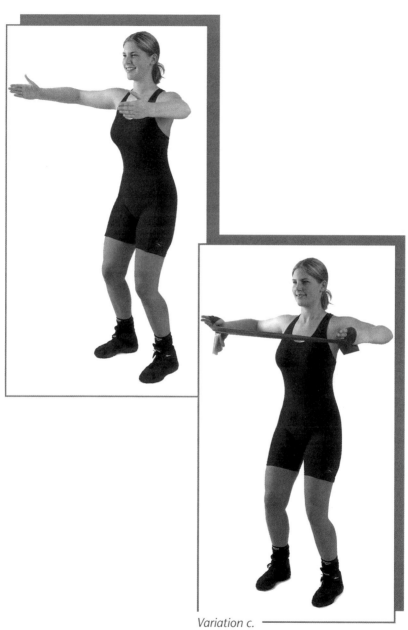

Variation c.

58 Strengthening exercise without equipment

TRAINING GOAL   **Strengthening** the shoulder girdle muscles
                       Strengthening the back muscles
                       Strengthening the latissimus dorsi

Description
Starting position: Take up the "basic deep torso bend position".
                       Hold your arms at the side of your body, your wrist are
                       bent downwards.
Exercise: Hold this position. Push your hands harder backwards.

Tips
- The tension between your shoulder blades increases, and your shoulder blades move together and pull downwards at the same time.
- *Point of awareness:* Keep your spine stable. Bend your torso as far forwards as possible while keeping it straight.
- Keep your cervical spine extended in line with your spine.
- Bend your legs.

Variations
a. Move your bent arms forwards, your thumbs point downwards. Pull on imaginary threads with your hands and move your elbows horizontally downwards to the floor.
b. As described in variation a., push your hands and lower arms slowly forwards under tension.
c. As described in variation b., hold an exercise band between your hands under slight tension.
d. As described, now, from the u-position bring one arm straight downwards and backwards, then forwards and upwards again. Imagine that you are pulling on a wire rope with weights, while you move your arm backwards under control and under tension.
e. As described in variation c., pull on an exercise band that you have attached to a wall bar or a door during the backwards movement of your arm.

difficulty
easy
medium
hard

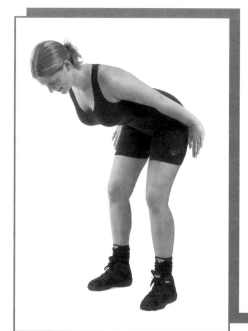

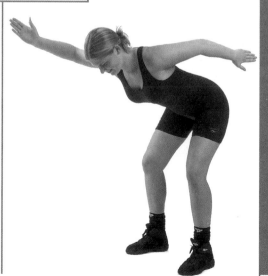

Variation d.

59 Strengthening exercise without equipment

TRAINING GOAL **Strengthening** the shoulder girdle muscles
Stabilising the whole trunk

Description
Starting position: Stand up straight with your feet hip-width apart with your back against a wall that is a good foot length away. Your coccygeal spine, your shoulder blades and the back of your head touch the wall. Place your arms by your sides with the backs of your hands against the wall.

Exercise: Press the backs of your hands against the wall.

Tips
■ Maintain contact between your head and your back and the wall, in spite of the increase in tension.
■ Continue breathing normally even during the increase in tension.

Variation
a. Press your hands together behind your back while standing up straight and maintaining a stable tension in your back.

difficulty
easy
medium
hard

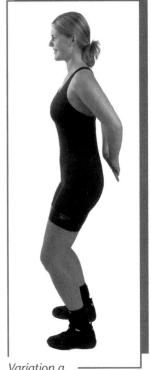

Variation a.

60 Strengthening exercise without equipment

TRAINING GOAL **Strengthening** the shoulder girdle muscles
Strengthening the back muscles

Description
Starting position: From the all fours position, change to the deep forward slide position.
Your arms are extended in line with your body; your weight is shifted backwards.
Exercise: Raise one straightened arm. Tilt your wrist slightly outwards.

Tips
▪▪ *Point of awareness:* Do not raise your upper body with your arm. Keep your spine stable, do not twist it.
▪▪ Keep your cervical spine extended in line with your spine.
▪▪ Continue to breathe evenly.

difficulty
easy
medium
hard

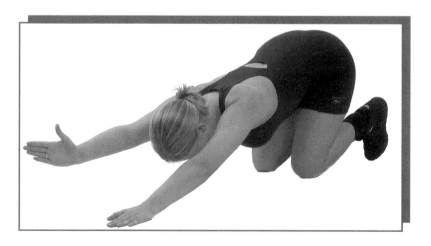

4   Exercises for the Abdominal Muscles

61 Strengthening exercise without equipment

TRAINING GOAL   **Strengthening** the rectus abdominis muscles.

Description
Starting position: Take up the "basic supine position". Raise your legs, feet flexed. Your hands are placed behind your head, supporting your head position, your elbows point out to the side.

Exercise: Raise your shoulder girdle and head from the floor. Keep your leg bent at right angles and alternately extend each leg forwards and upwards.

Tips
▬ Keep your cervical spine extended.
▬ Keep your lumbar spine in contact with the floor.
▬ Vary the direction of the leg extension, sometimes diagonally forwards and upwards, sometimes horizontal to the floor.

difficulty
easy
medium
hard

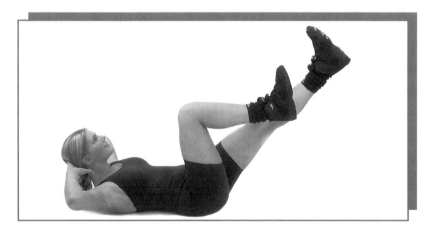

62 Strengthening exercise without equipment

TRAINING GOAL — **Strengthening** the rectus abdominis muscles

Description

Starting position: Take up the "basic supine position". Keep your legs extended with your feet flexed. Your arms are stretched out behind your head.

Exercise: Raise your shoulder girdle, head and arms from the floor. Bring your hand diagonally towards your bent knee and increase the pressure there.

Tips
- Keep your head in line with your spine.
- Carry out the movement slowly and under control.
- Maintain contact between your lumbar spine and the floor throughout.

Variation
a. As described, but support your head with one hand.

difficulty
easy
medium
hard

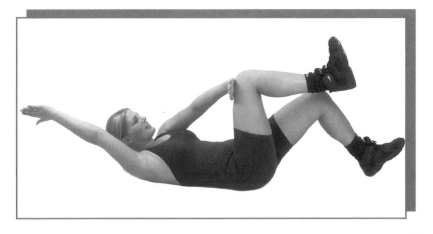

113

63 Strengthening exercise without equipment and with a partner

TRAINING GOAL | Partner 1:Strengthening the rectus abdominis muscles
Partner 2: Strengthening the back extensor muscles

Exercise situation: | Both partners carry out different exercises.

Description

Starting position: | Take up the "basic supine position" with your knees bent.
Partner 2 sits with their back straight in front of you.

Exercise: | Sit up slowly and tap your partner between their shoulder blades.

Tips

- Keep your neck straight.
- Straighten your body from your sternum upwards.
- Your partner tilts their pelvis forwards so that they can sit upright. Otherwise, they can support themselves with both hands behind their back, to help them sit up straight.

difficulty
easy
medium
hard

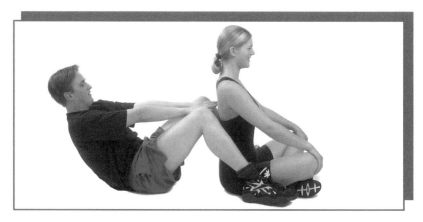

64 Strengthening exercise without equipment

TRAINING GOAL   Strengthening the lower abdominal muscles

Description
Starting position: Take up the "basic supine position". Keep your legs bent and flex your feet. Your hands are placed behind your head, supporting the head position, your elbows point out to the sides.

Exercise: Try to raise your bottom from the floor and push it forwards.

Tips
■ Keep your thighs perpendicular and push your knees upwards.
■ Always work in an upwards direction. Even if you do not raise your pelvis from the floor, just trying to do this has a strengthening effect.
■ To begin with, let your head and shoulders stay relaxed on the floor.
■ Breathe evenly throughout.

difficulty
easy
medium
hard

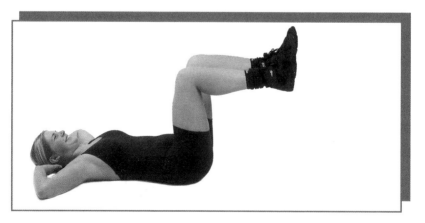

65 Strengthening exercise without equipment

TRAINING GOAL   **Strengthening** the oblique abdominal muscles

Description
Starting position: Take up the "basic supine position".
                        Bend your legs, straighten your arms and hold them
                        above your head.
Exercise: Raise your head and shoulder girdle from the floor.
                        Push the palms of your hands upwards alternately.

Tips
■ Carry out the movement symmetrically and under control.
■ Hold your head in line with your body.
■ *Point of awareness:* Raise each shoulder with the respective arm, so
  bringing your shoulder towards the opposite side of the pelvis.
■ Your sternum faces upwards. Avoid rounding your back.

difficulty
easy
medium
hard

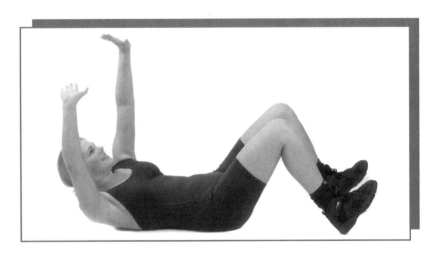

66 Strengthening exercise without equipment

TRAINING GOAL   **Strengthening** the oblique abdominal muscles

Description
Starting position: Take up the "basic supine position". Bend your legs and flex your feet. Your hands are placed behind your head and support your head position, your elbows point out to the side.

Exercise: Press with a flat hand against your opposite knee, so creating tension.
Your shoulder girdle turns towards your knee.

Tips
▬▬ Keep your head in line with your spine.
▬▬ Pull your sternum upwards. Avoid rounding your spine.
▬▬ Breathe evenly throughout.

difficulty
easy
medium
hard

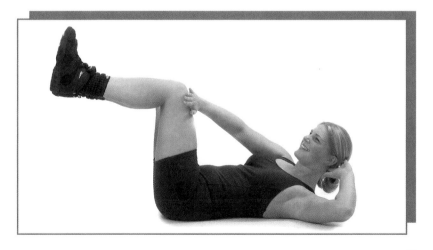

67 Strengthening exercise without equipment

TRAINING GOAL   Strengthening the oblique abdominal muscles

Description

Starting position: Take up the "basic supine position". Bend one leg, straighten the other and point it upwards. Flex your feet. Your hands are placed behind your head and support the head position, your elbows point right out to the side.

Exercise: Raise your head and shoulder girdle from the floor. Move your straight leg to the side towards the floor. Keep your pelvis stable.

Tips

▪ Do not turn your pelvis.
▪ In the beginning, you can let your head and shoulder girdle remain relaxed on the floor.

difficulty

easy
medium
hard

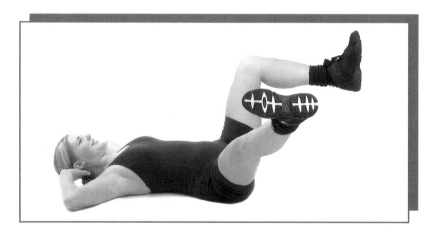

68 Strengthening exercise without equipment

TRAINING GOAL **Strengthening** the rectus abdominis muscles

Description
Starting position: Stand up straight with your feet hip-width apart.
Push your arms downwards, with your wrists bent.
Exercise: Place one foot forwards; heel down. Lean your body backwards.
Push the opposite arm to the extended leg upwards, with bent wrist.

Tips
- Your upper palm pushes upwards, your fingertips point inwards and your elbows outwards.
- *Point of awareness:* Maintain the tension in your trunk in particular, by stretching the abdominal and buttock muscles. Avoid overstretching the spine and hollowing your back.

difficulty
easy
medium
hard

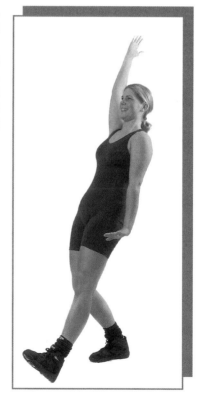

69 Strengthening exercise without equipment

TRAINING GOAL **Strengthening** the rectus abdominis muscles

Description

Starting position: Sit up straight on a stool.
Spread your fingers, lay your hands so that the palm of one is on your stomach and the back of the other is on your lumbar spine.

Exercise: Lean your upper body backwards.

Tips
- Keep your back actively upright. Move only by bending and stretching your hips backwards and forwards.
- Keep your neck extended in line with your spine.
- Use your hands to feel that you are keeping your upper body stable.

Variations
a. When leaning backwards, raise your legs from the floor and keep them raised at right angles.
b. Push both arms straight downwards near your body. Bend your wrists, so that your fingers point forwards.
c. As described in variations a. and b., in addition bring the arms alternately straight upwards in line with the line of the side of the body. Make sure that your trunk is stable throughout.

difficulty
easy
medium
hard

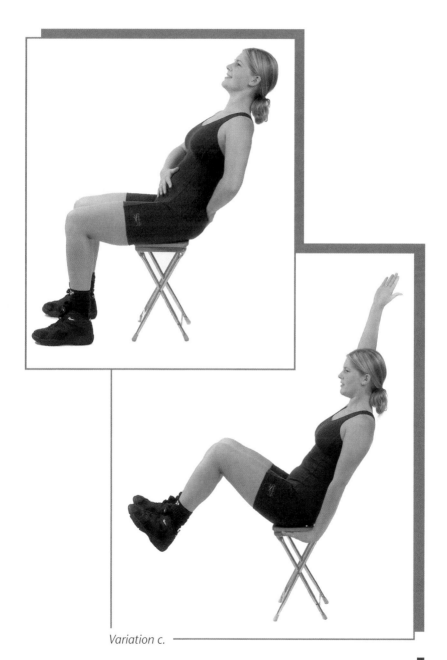

Variation c.

5 Exercises for the Buttock and Leg Muscles

70 Strengthening exercise without equipment

TRAINING GOAL **Strengthening** the gluteus maximus
Strengthening the gluteus medius and gluteus minimus
Stabilising the lumbar spine-hip area

Description
Starting position: Lie on your back on the floor.
Bend your legs; your arms are straight behind your head on the floor, the palms of your hands face upwards.

Exercise: Raise only your bottom up to your lumbar spine and roll up from the floor in a narrow arc.

Tips
■ *Point of awareness:* only roll up your lumbar spine. Keep your thoracic spine in contact with the floor. Imagine that by rolling up your stomach, you are bringing your pubic bone nearer to your sternum.
■ In the described movement, your lumbar spine is flat to slightly round.
■ In the beginning, you can keep your arms lying by your sides. Then use your arms as support.
■ Avoid letting your pelvis sag on one side, which could make your lumbar spine twist.

Variations
a. Hold your arms crossed in front of your chest, pulling your elbows out slightly to the side.
b. Pull the tips of your toes towards you and press your heels to the floor.
c. As described in a. and b, in addition, straighten one leg and raise it from the floor. Your thighs are both at the same height. Keep your feet flexed.

difficulty
easy
medium
hard

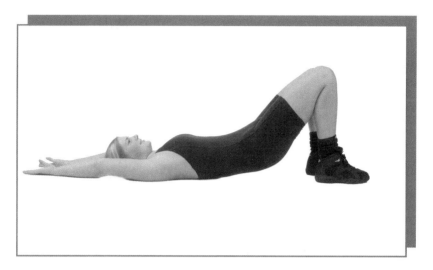

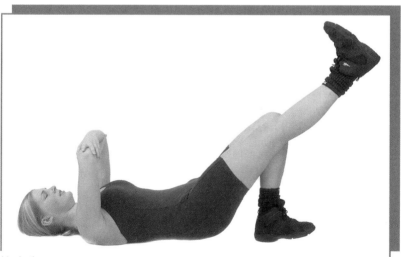

Variation c.

71 Strengthening exercise without equipment

TRAINING GOAL **Strengthening** the gluteus maximus
Stablising the lumbar spine - hip area

Description

Starting position: Lie on your back on the floor.
Bend your legs and pull in your feet. Your arms lie on the floor at the side of your body, the palms of your hands face upwards.

Exercise: Roll up your spine beginning at your bottom, slowly until the complete extension of your hips on the floor.

Tips

■ Hold the hip stretch for a few seconds, before laying your back and bottom vertebra by vertebra on the floor once more.
■ Your thighs are in line with your body.
■ Avoid tilting your pelvis to one side when raising your legs.

Variations

a. Walk on the spot, without lowering your bottom.
b. Raise your hands and arms from the floor.
c. Place your heels further away from your body. Flex your feet. Avoid over-extending your spine, though. This will bring your bottom nearer the floor when your hips are extended.
d. As described in variation c., in addition alternately raise one leg from the floor.

difficulty

easy
medium
hard

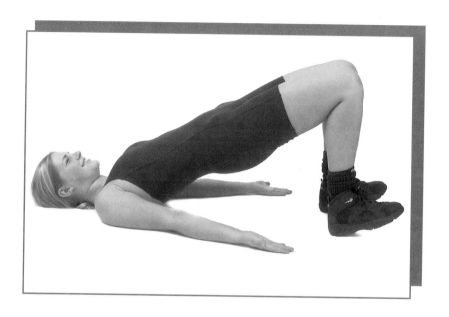

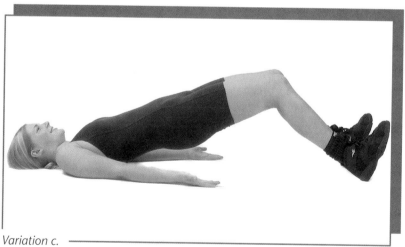

Variation c.

72 Strengthening exercise without equipment

TRAINING GOAL

Strengthening the gluteus maximus
Stabilising the lumbar spine - hip area

Description
Starting position: Lie on your back on the floor.
Bend your legs and flex your feet. Your arms lie by your sides, the palms of your hands facing upwards. Extend one leg upwards.

Exercise: Roll your spine starting from the bottom off the floor, until your hips are completely extended.

Tips
- Hold the hip extension for a few seconds, before laying your back and bottom vertebra by vertebra under control onto the floor again.
- Avoid letting your hips drop on one side, which could make your spine turn to the side.
- Flex both feet, in order to improve pelvic stability.

difficulty
easy
medium
hard

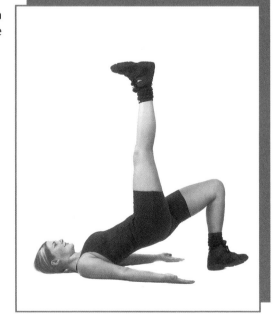

73 Strengthening exercise without equipment

TRAINING GOAL   **Strengthening** the gluteus maximus
Stabilising the lumbar spine - hip area

Description
Starting position: Lie on your back on the floor.
Bend your legs and flex your feet. Your arms lie at your sides, the palms of your hands facing upwards.
Exercise: Roll up your spine slowly off the floor, beginning from the buttocks until the hips are completely extended. Now bring one bent leg towards the upper body and press the knee against your hands.

Tips
▧ Hold the tension during the hip extension for a few seconds.
▧ Avoid letting your pelvis drop to one side.

difficulty
easy
medium
hard

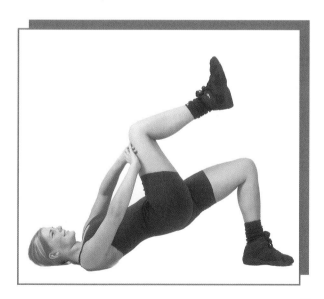

74 Strengthening exercise without equipment

TRAINING GOAL   **Strengthening** the gluteus minimus
Strengthening the lateral torso muscles
Stabilising the pelvis

Description

Starting position: Take up the "basic side lying position".
Extend the top leg.

Exercise: Raise and lower the extended top leg.

Tips

- *Point of awareness:* Bring the straight leg up high, your heel pushed well back. Only then will you strengthen the buttock muscles and stabilize your pelvis.
- Place your head on your outstretched arm to support your neck.
- The bent bottom leg provides increased pelvic stability. Avoid evasive action in the pelvis.

Variations

a. As described, bend the straightened leg at the knee in the high position, before straightening it and bringing it down to the floor again.

b. As described, bring the leg from the high rear position downwards and forwards. Tap your heel just in front of the leg on the floor, before straightening it and bringing it backwards and upwards again.
In this way, the gluteus minimus muscles are alternately strengthened by raising the straightened leg, and stretched by lowering the bent leg.

difficulty

easy
medium
hard

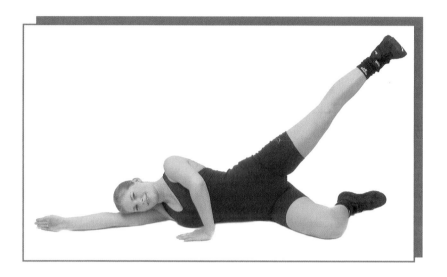

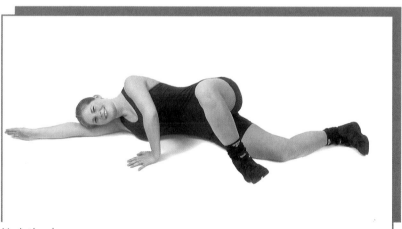

Variation b.

75 Strengthening exercise without equipment

TRAINING GOAL · · · · · · · **Strengthening** the gluteus maximus
Strengthening the inner thigh muscles

Description
Starting position: · · · Take up the "basic side lying position".
Bend the top leg and place it over the bottom leg.
Exercise: · · · · · · · · · · · Move the bottom, straight, leg up and down, without
touching the floor.

Tips
- Carry out the movement slowly and under control
- Avoid evasive action in the pelvis; keep it stable.
- Lay your head on your outstretched arm to relax your cervical spine.

difficulty
easy
medium
hard

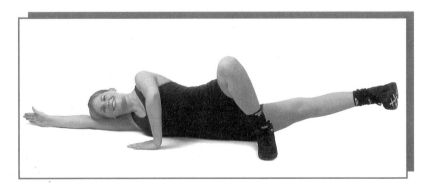

76 Strengthening exercise without equipment

TRAINING GOAL **Strengthening** the quadriceps muscles
Strengthening the hip extensor muscles
Stabilising the whole trunk

Description
Starting position: Sit up straight on a stool.
Exercise: Straighten and raise one leg, with your foot flexed.
Pull your leg further upwards by an imaginary thread
with the opposite hand.

Tips
▬ *Point of awareness:* Straighten and raise one leg, with your foot
flexed. Straighten your spine. Avoid rounding your back. Lift your leg
to a height where you can keep your back straight.
▬ Keep your neck erect.

Variation
a. You can also carry out the exercise sitting up straight on the floor.
Make sure your back posture is correct.

difficulty
easy
medium
hard

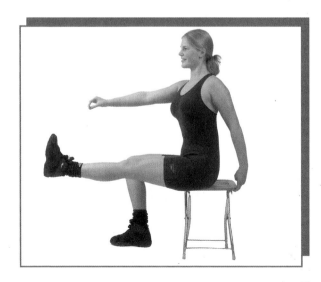

77 Strengthening exercise without equipment with a partner

TRAINING GOAL   **Strengthening** the quadriceps muscles
Strengthening the shoulder blade muscles

Description
Starting position: Stand back to back, bending your knees slightly. Push
the backs of your hands together beside your bodies.
Exercise: Bend and stretch your knees in unison, while pressing
your hands gently together.

Tips
▬ Your backs are relaxed.

Variation
a. Interlink your arms. Your backs
remain straight.

difficulty
easy
medium
hard

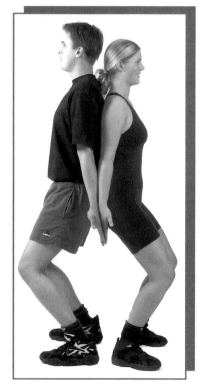

6 Exercises for Back and Trunk Stability

78 Stabilising exercise without equipment

TRAINING GOAL   **Stabilising** the whole trunk
                       Strengthening the abdominal muscles

Description
Starting position: Take up the "basic all fours position".
Exercise: Raise both knees slightly from the floor, keeping your
                       back stable.

Tips
- Hold this position.
- Keep your cervical spine extended, look at the floor.
- *Point of awareness:* Keep your spine stable and your back in its physiological shape.

Variation
a. walk on the spot with your knees raised.

difficulty
easy
medium
hard

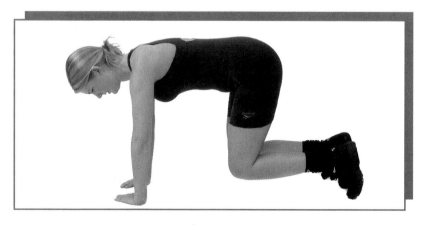

79 Stabilising exercise without equipment

TRAINING GOAL   **Stabilising** the whole trunk
Strengthening the abdominal muscles

Description
Starting position: Lie on the floor on your stomach, supported by your lower arms. Your elbows are under your shoulder joints. Flex your feet.
Exercise: Raise your pelvis from the floor with your knees bent, until your back is in a horizontal position.

Tips
■ Keep your back stable.
■ Keep your cervical spine in line with your spine.
■ Lay your hands perpendicularly on the floor.
■ Place a flat cushion under your knees.

Variations
a. Raise one leg straight until it is horizontal to the floor. Keep your heel pushed back.
b. Lift one arm from the floor and bring it straight forwards. Keep the palm of your hand perpendicular and tilt your wrist slightly outwards. Your thumb points upwards. Be careful not to let your shoulder girdle drop to the side. Your neck remains extended.

difficulty
easy
medium
hard

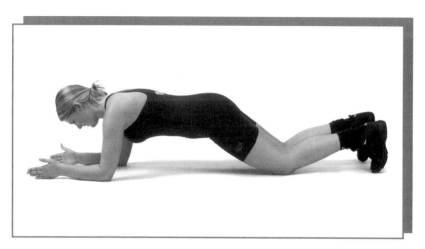

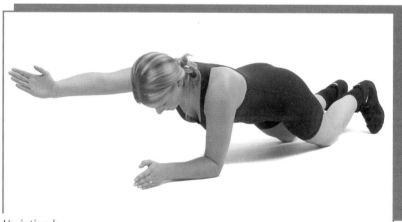

Variation b.

135

80 Stabilising exercise without equipment

TRAINING GOAL   **Stabilising** the whole trunk
                       Strengthening the abdominal muscles

Description
Starting position: Lie on your stomach, supported by your lower arms.
                       Your elbows are below your shoulder joints. Flex your
                       feet.
Exercise: Extend your hips and your knees.

Tips
▬ Keep your back stable.
▬ *Point of awareness:* avoid "sagging" in the pelvic area, and a
  "potbelly" for physiologically effective training. A sagging pelvis leads
  to hollowing of the back and an increased load on the lumbar spine,
  raising the bottom decreases the activity and the strengthening of the
  abdominal muscles, by diminishing the lever. In comparison with the
  hollowing, a raised bottom with a stable and straight back is not
  damaging, in terms of physiological loading.
▬ Keep your cervical spine in line with your spine.
▬ Place your hands perpendicular to the floor.
▬ If you have trouble with this exercise, do the two preceding exercises
  first to begin with.

Variations
a. Raise one leg straight until it is horizontal to the floor. Keep your heel
   pushed back.
b. As described in variation a., raise one leg after the other and place
   them in the straddle position, thereby making the exercise even more
   difficult.
c. Walk on the spot.
d. Raise one arm from the floor and bring it straight forwards. Keep the
   palm of your hand perpendicular and tilt your wrist slightly outwards.
   Your thumb points upwards.

difficulty
easy
medium
hard

136

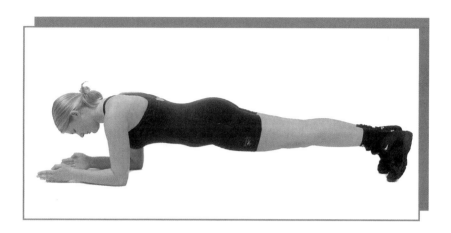

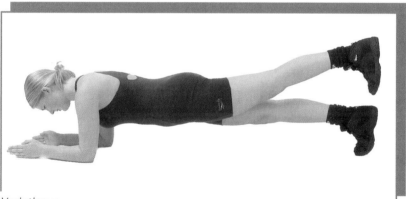

Variation a.

81 Stabilising exercise without equipment

TRAINING GOAL   **Stabilising** the whole trunk
Strengthening the lateral trunk muscles

Description
Starting position: Take up the "basic side lying position".
Support yourself on your underarm. Your elbow is
beneath your shoulder.
Exercise: Straighten your hips and knees, until your upper body
and thighs form a line. Extend your top arm along
the side of your body, with your wrist bent
downwards, your fingers point forwards.

Tips
■ Your head, your pelvis and your heels are in a line.
■ Keep your hips straight and do not let your pelvis sink.

Variation
a. As described, place your top leg straight in front of the bottom leg, and
extend your body. Flex your feet.

difficulty
easy
medium
hard

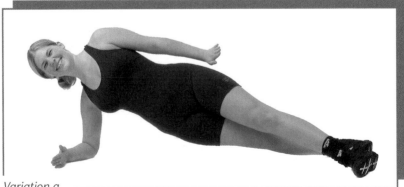

Variation a.

82 Stabilising exercise without equipment with a partner

TRAINING GOAL   **Stabilising** the whole trunk
Strengthening the abdominal musculature

Exercise situation: Both partners carry out the same exercises together.

Description
Starting position: Both take up the "basic all fours position".
Exercise: Push your bottoms together with the same pressure.
Key concept: "Together we are strong!"

Tips
▬ Maintain the tension in your stomach.
▬ Stabilise your whole body. Support yourself with your arms.

Variations
a. Try to push each other away.
b. Stand next to each other and push against each other with your shoulders and hips.

difficulty
easy
medium
hard

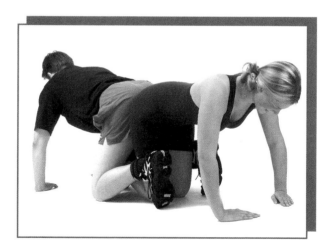

139

83 Stabilising exercise without equipment with a partner

TRAINING GOAL   Partner 1: **Stabilising** the whole torso
                       Improving the extension of the spine
                       Partner 2: **Strengthening** the back muscles

Exercise situation: One partner provides support and assistence; the other is manually stretched.

Description
Starting position: Sit up straight with your legs apart.
                        Your partner stands behind you.
Exercise: Your partner stretches your spine by pulling your hands.

Tips
▬ Keep your cervical spine erect.
▬ Keep your bottom on the floor.
▬ Sit upright at all times. From there you can move your legs together or cross your legs, or put a cushion under your bottom, if this makes it easier for you to sit with your back straight.
▬ Your partner keeps his back stable and tenses mainly the lower trunk muscles.
▬ After the stretch, roll down your spine and let it hang a little, and breathe in hard to relax your back.

Variation
Exercise situation: Both partners carry out the same exercise together.
a. Sit on the floor back to back in the straddle position. Bring your arms slightly outwards and point them upwards. Hold your partner's hands or lower arms and stretch them slowly upwards.
   You can either stretch together or one after the other.
   Key concept: "Pulling each other makes us more flexible".

difficulty
easy
medium
hard

140

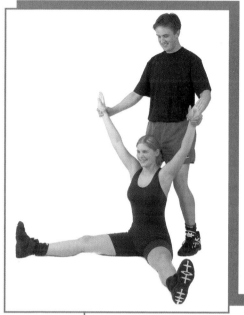

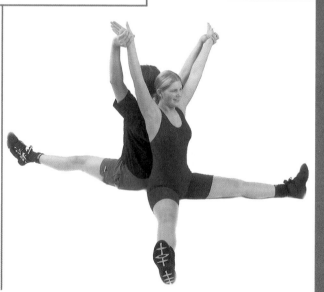

Variation a.

84 Stabilising exercise without equipment with a partner

TRAINING GOAL   **Stabilising** the whole trunk
                   Strengthening the back muscles

Exercise situation: Both partners carry out the same exercise together.

Description
Starting position: Sit up straight back-to-back on the floor in the
                        straddle position.
Exercise: Hold your arms out to the sides and push the backs of
                        your hands together.

Tips
■ Try to keep your distance from each other and not to touch each other.
   Key concept: "A crack is visible between your backs!"
■ Stretch your cervical spine and your whole trunk upwards.

Variations
a. Also carry out the exercise sitting on a stool or standing up.
b. *Without a partner:* Carry out the exercise alone against a wall.

difficulty
easy
medium
hard

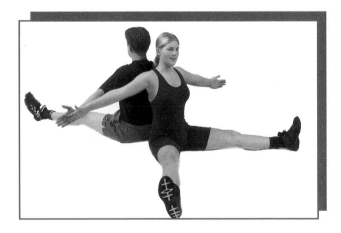

85 Stabilising exercise without equipment with a partner

TRAINING GOAL

Partner 1: **Stabilising** the whole trunk.
Partner 2: **Strengthening** the torso muscles

Exercise situation:

One partner carries out the exercise, the other supports.

Description

Starting position:

Stand up straight with your feet hip-width apart.
Your partner stands behind you.

Exercise:

While you keep your trunk stable by tensing your muscles, your partner tries to destabilise you by applying pressure points to different parts of your back.

Tips

■ Resist your partner's pressure with concentration and relaxation. Stabilise your body so well that it does not move.

■ Your partner tries to apply the pressure points mainly diagonally to each other. He builds up the pressure continuously, not in jerky movements.

difficulty
easy
medium
hard

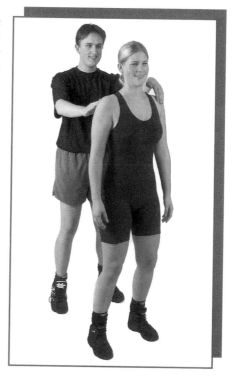

86 Stabilising exercise without equipment with a partner

TRAINING GOAL	**Stabilising** the whole trunk **Strengthening** the back muscles
Exercise situation:	Both partners carry out the same exercise together.

Description

Starting position: Stand up straight with your feet shoulder-width apart. Your knees are slightly bent. Join your hands and stretch your arms forwards. The backs of your hands touch on one side.

Exercise: Press your hands together.

Tips
- Tense your trunk muscles before pressing your hands together.
- Keep your pelvis, shoulder girdle and trunk stable; do not turn your torso.
- Push only so strongly that you can both maintain the starting position.

Variations
a. **Without a partner:** Carry out the exercise alone against the wall or against a doorframe.
b. Vary the height of your hands, from the navel to the head. In this way you also vary the intensity of trunk strength needed to remain stable in the starting position.
c. Stand in the starting position and place the palms of your hands low and high to the sides at a diagonal. If necessary, change your foot position from the parallel position to the stride position to achieve better trunk stability.

difficulty
easy
medium
hard

144

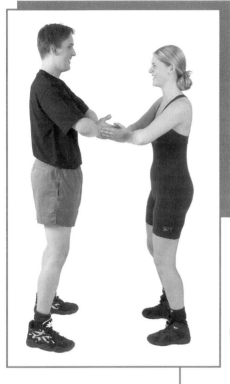

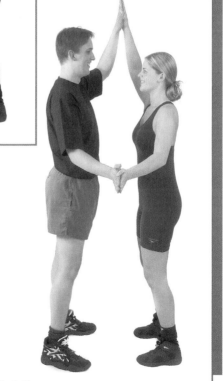

Variation c.

87 Stabilising exercise without equipment with a partner

TRAINING GOAL   **Stabilising** the whole trunk
        Strengthening the back muscles
        Strengthening the quadriceps muscles

Exercise situation: Both partners carry out the same exercise together.

Description
Starting position: Both stand in the stride position with a stable trunk,
        the upper bodies lean forwards towards each other.
Exercise: Push the palms of your right hands together, your
        elbows point outwards. At the same time, push your
        left arms downwards and backwards with your wrist
        tilted forwards.

Tips
■ Tense your trunk muscles firmly in your stomach and bottom.
■ Transfer your weight mainly onto your front leg. Your rear leg remains
 straight; your heels push backwards and downwards.

difficulty
easy
medium
hard

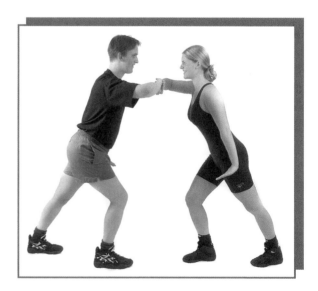

VI Strength Exercises with an Exercise Bar – a Classic Aid to Effective Training

Themes
■ The exercise bar as an effective exercise tool
■ Static strengthening and stabilising exercises
■ Stabilising exercises alone or in pairs

Focus
The variety and effectiveness that the simple exercise bar can offer are the main benefits when training for muscle strength and joint stability. The exercises carried out are mainly static. They are therefore often held for some time or carried out slowly and under control.

In any case, try to take up the correct starting position for each exercise, with the correct foot position. Then load yourself as heavily as necessary during the exercise, but only as much as possible. You can very easily determine and vary your own loading strength with the bar using your individual judgement.

Requirements
■ An upright and active standing position.
■ The deliberate stabilising of the whole spine and the trunk.
■ Gain familiarity with the bar by simple catching and gripping exercises.
■ The safe and full grip of the bar.
■ The complementary mobility exercises.

1 The Special Features of Training with the Bar

Despite its simplicity, the exercise bar can be a versatile training tool that is suitable not only for the training session, but also for example for warming up. The bar is a rigid exercise tool. They are usually 80 – 100 cm long, the longer length being recommended for adults.

It can be easily substituted when exercising at home. Use a broom handle for example, or alternatively a small hand towel. This should be held at the ends like a bar, and pulled by the hands to bring it under tension. In this way, it gives way very little, which makes the pull outwards with the hands clearly noticeable – substantially better then the bar.

Take care that the bar does not fall. In particular, in the throwing or reaction exercises, you must take care that your feet are not hit by the falling bar.

The Exercise Principles

Along with the exercise principles of general functional strengthening exercises, as described in chapter V, the following features also apply to exercising with the bar:

- Pay attention to the recommended hand grip when carrying out the exercises: be aware that in particular the kind of grip – whether from above or from below – affects the stretching and extending of the spine. In particular choose the grip that turns your shoulders outwards. You will stand up straighter like this. Often the grip of the bar is from below.
- Keep your trunk and spine stable by tensing the large trunk muscles, i.e. stomach, pelvis, buttocks and back muscles.
- Pull the ends of the bar outwards with your hands or push them centrally back together (carry out only horizontal and vertical bar movements, but combine these with the lateral pulling and pushing direction in alternation).

Be particularly careful in the static exercises to continue to breathe naturally and evenly (do not hold your breath!). The danger of holding your breath is greater in static exercises with high muscle tension than in dynamic exercises.

2 Exercises

88 Strengthening exercise with a bar

TRAINING GOAL   **Strengthening** the back and arm muscles
Strengthening the shoulder blade muscles
Awareness of the erect spinal posture

Description
Starting position: Stand up straight with your feet shoulder-width apart. Hold the bar with your elbows at right angles at shoulder height in front of the body.
Exercise: Pull the bar outwards and move it forwards.
Push the bar together and move it back towards your chest.

Tips
■ Maintain the tension in the lower torso; your stomach and buttock muscles are tensed.

Variation
a. Change the grip: hold the bar from above and from underneath.

difficulty
easy
medium
hard

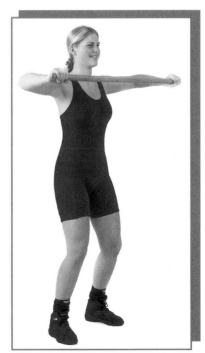

149

89 Strengthening exercise with a bar

Training Goal

Strengthening the back and arm muscles
Strengthening the shoulder blade muscles
Awareness of the spinal posture

Description

Starting position: Stand up straight with your feet shoulder-width apart. Hold the bar with your elbows at right angles at shoulder height in front of the body.

Exercise: Turn to the side with your pelvis stable and your shoulder girdle firm.

Tips

- Move under control and slowly during the rotation of your spine.Do not twist your body. Do not tilt to the side.
- At the farthest point of your shoulder girdle turn, you can move your head a little further to the side.

Variation

a. Turn your forward-facing upper body and shoulder girdle to the side. Your pelvis remains stable and does not move.

difficulty

easy
medium
hard

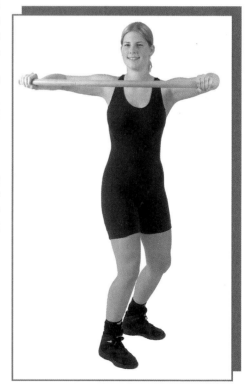

90 Strengthening exercise with a bar

Training Goal **Strengthening** the back and arm muscles
Strengthening the shoulder blade muscles

Description
Starting position: Stand up straight with your feet shoulder-width apart. Hold the bar above your head.
Exercise: Bend your upper body with a firm shoulder girdle and stable arm carriage to the side. Your pelvis remains stable.

Tips
■■ Move your elbows backwards until you build up tension between the shoulder blades. Maintain the muscular tension in your lower trunk.

difficulty
easy
medium
hard

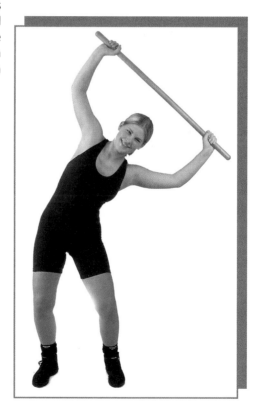

91 Strengthening exercise with a bar

TRAINING GOAL   **Strengthening** the back and arm muscles
                    Strengthening the shoulder blade muscles

Description
Starting position: Stand up straight with your feet shoulder-width apart.
                        Hold the bar with your elbows at right angles above
                        your head.
Exercise: Pull the bar outwards and move it upwards.
                        Push the bar together and move it back to the starting
                        position.

Tips
■■ Maintain the tension in the lower trunk; your stomach and buttock
muscles are tensed.
■■ Move the bar in a perpendicular plane behind your head upwards and
backwards. This stretches your spine, your elbows move slightly
backwards.

Variations
a. Combine this exercise with exercise 89.
b. Change your foot and leg position to the stride position. Lean your
upper body forwards, so that your body forms a line from your head to
your rear heel. Now, as described, move the bar from the inclined
position forwards and upwards in the diagonal and back behind your
head backwards again.
Change your foot position.
c. As described in variation b. move the bar at shoulder height
horizontally to the floor in front of your body and backwards again.

difficulty
easy
medium
hard

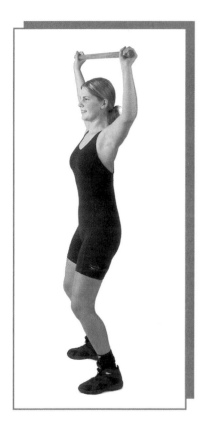

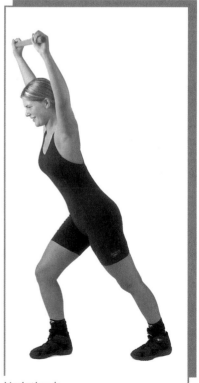

Variation b.

153

92 Strengthening exercise with a bar and with a partner

TRAINING GOAL   **Strengthening** the back muscles
                     Strengthening the biceps muscles
                     Strengthening the erect body posture

Exercise situation: One partner carries out the exercise and the other
                        supports.

Description
Starting position: Sit with your legs slightly bent in front of your partner
                        and hold the bar horizontally with both hands above
                        your head. Your partner stands behind you and grips
                        the bar from below.
Exercise: Now try to pull the bar towards your shoulders
                        against your partner's resistance.

Tips
- Tense your stomach muscles slightly to stabilise your trunk.
- Sit up as straight as possible, and do not let your upper body sag.
- Your partner stands firm with his feet in the split position.
- Your partner keeps his spine stable.
- If necessary, your partner can press the outside of his leg against your
  upright back, in order to support your back posture.

Variations
a. Push the bar upwards against your partner's resistance, and then pull it
   back down to the starting position.
b. Move the bar from the starting position in a quarter turn against the
   resistance of your partner forwards and downwards. Finish the turn at
   shoulder height. Then bring the bar back again above your head
   against your partner's resistance.
c. Your partner deliberately varies the resistance that he provides to your
   movement.

difficulty
easy
medium
hard

154

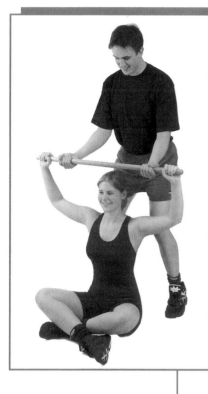

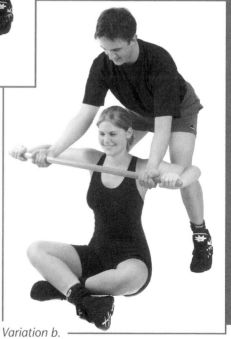

Variation b.

93 Strengthening exercise with a bar

| TRAINING GOAL | **Strengthening** the back muscles |
| | **Strengthening** the shoulder blade muscles |

Description

Starting position:	Take up the "basic prone position".
	Grip the bar from above with both hands and hold it above your bottom.
Exercise:	Push the ends of the bar together while straightening your upper body.

Tips

- Your neck always remains in line with your spine, look at the floor. Be aware of the tension between your shoulder blades.
- Be careful to breathe calmly and evenly.
- Tense your stomach and buttock muscles, and straighten your pelvis.
- Your spine remains neutral throughout.

Variations

a. Pull the ends of the bar apart.
b. Move the bar further above your bottom.
c. Grip the bar with bent arms in the u-position. Pull the ends of the bar apart and stretch your arms slowly forwards until they are horizontal to the floor. Then push the bar together and move your arms slowly back to the starting position.
d. As described in variation c., move your arms further backwards and downwards, while moving the bar back over the back of your head.
e. As described in variation c., push the bar sideways, with stable arms.

difficulty

easy
medium
hard

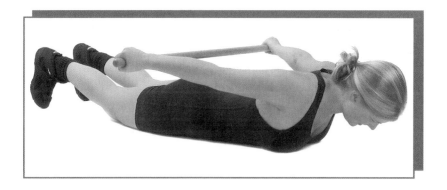

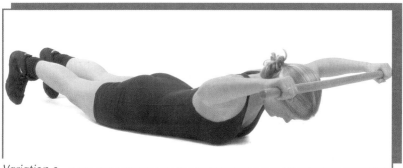

Variation c.

94 Strengthening exercise with a bar

TRAINING GOAL   **Strengthening** the back and arm muscles
                       Strengthening the shoulder blade muscles
                       Awareness of spinal posture

Description
Starting position: Stand up straight with your feet shoulder-width apart.
                        Hold the bar along your spine.
Exercise: Pull the ends of the bar apart.

Tips
■ Your cervical spine remains directly in line with the rest of your spine, look horizontally at the floor. Do you have the feeling that you are growing taller?
■ Be aware of the tension between your shoulder blades.
■ Ensure that you breathe calmly and evenly.
■ Tense your stomach and buttock muscles, straighten your pelvis.
■ Avoid a backwards over-extension of your trunk (hollowing your back).
■ Keep your knees slightly bent. Do not straighten your arms completely.

Variations
a. Push the ends of the bar together.
b. Move the bar slowly up and down your spine.
c. As described, pull the bar diagonally over your spine.
d. Hold the bar horizontally to the floor; grip it from below so that your shoulders are turned outwards. Now push the ends of the bar together. Maintain the tension in your shoulders and trunk.
e. As described in variation d., pull the ends of the bar together.

difficulty
easy
medium
hard

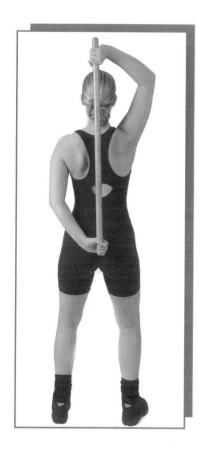

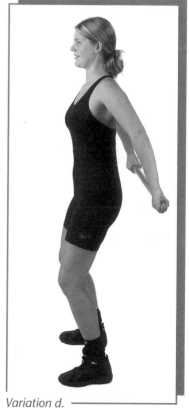

Variation d.

95 Strengthening exercise with a bar

TRAINING GOAL **Strengthening** the back muscles
Strengthening the shoulder blade muscles
Awareness of spinal posture

Description
Starting position: Stand up straight with your feet shoulder-width apart. Grip the bar from below. Hold it at navel height in front of your body.
Exercise: Pull the ends of the bar apart and push them together alternately.

Tips
- ■ Bend your legs slightly. Make sure that your legs are correctly in line.
- ■ Be aware of the tension between your shoulder blades.
- ■ Avoid hollowing your back by keeping your lower trunk muscles firmly tensed.

Variations
a. As described, begin the exercise at shoulder height with nearly straight arms.
b. Bend deeper at your knees while pushing your knees outwards over your feet.
c. Combine the separate variations with the basic exercise in a continuous exercise.

difficulty
easy
medium
hard

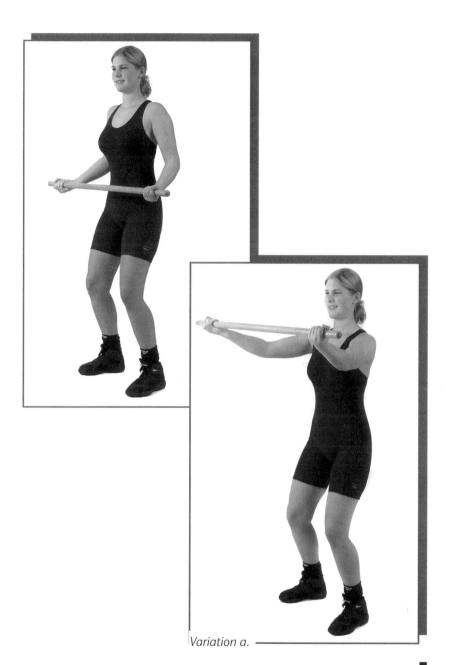

Variation a.

96 Strengthening exercise with a bar

TRAINING GOAL   **Strengthening** the back extensor muscles
                  Strengthening the abdominal muscles
                  Awareness of the spinal posture

Description
Starting position: Sit up straight.
                       Grip the bar from below. Hold it in front of your body.
Exercise: Push the ends of the bar apart to get your spine in a
                       straight position.

Tips
▰ Extend your cervical spine.
▰ Tilt your pelvis forwards and extend your lumbar spine upwards.
▰ Continue to breathe and adapt your breathing cycle to the movement.

Variations
a. Push the ends of the bar together.
b. Begin from a relaxed position with a rounded back. Now pull on the
    ends of the bar while straightening your back.
Exercise situation: Both partners carry out the same exercise together.
c. Sit opposite each other and both hold the bar at right- angles to your
    bodies. Pull the ends of the bar apart and maintain the tension in your
    torsos.
d. As described in variation c., but straighten your upper body and round
    your back. While you carry out this exercise, your partner maintains the
    basic tension and sits up straight.

difficulty
easy
medium
hard

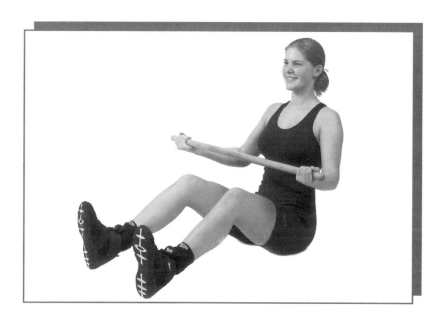

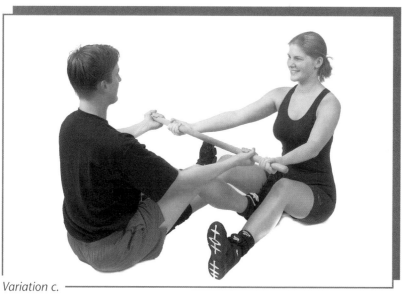

Variation c.

97 Strengthening exercise with a bar

TRAINING GOAL   **Strengthening** the shoulder girdle muscles
Strengthening the wide back muscles

Description

Starting position: Take up the "basic deep torso bend position".   Hold the bar in the u-position in front of your head.

Exercise: Pull the ends of the bar apart and push it both forwards and backwards.

Tips

■ Your cervical spine is straight.
■ The tension between your shoulder blades increases, as your shoulder blades move together and simultaneously pull downwards.
■ *Point of awareness:* Keep your spine stable. Only bend so far forwards so that you can keep your back straight.
■ Bend your legs.

difficulty

easy
medium
hard

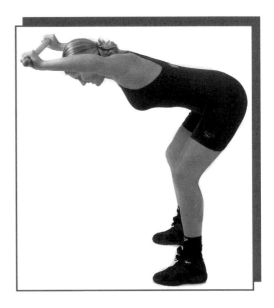

98 Strengthening exercise with a bar

TRAINING GOAL **Strengthening** the shoulder girdle muscles
Strengthening the back extensor muscles
Strengthening the front thigh muscles

Description

Starting position: Take up the "basic straight back bent position".
Grip the bar from below. Hold it in front of your body.

Exercise: Carry out the following continuous exercise sequence:
Lay the bar on the floor, stand up, bend down again,
lift the stick up and come back to the starting
position.

Tips

▬▬ Take care to adopt the physiologically correct back posture while
performing the exercise. Take up the correct basic positions such as
the straight-backed bent-over position and the upright standing
position.

difficulty
easy
medium
hard

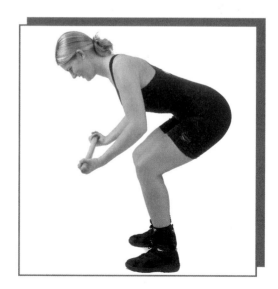

99 Strengthening exercise with a bar

Training Goal **Strengthening** the shoulder girdle muscles
Strengthening the back extensor muscles

Description
Starting position: Take up the "basic kneeling position".
Grip the bar from below and hold it under your bottom.
Exercise: Lean your upper body forwards. Pull the ends of the bar outwards.

Tips
▬ Keep your trunk stable; your spine remains straight.
▬ Move only by bending forwards from your hips.

Variations
a. Vary the pressure against your bottom and the pull on the bar while carrying out the exercise.
b. Pull the bar by bending your arms backwards past your bottom, then upwards and then back to the starting position.

difficulty
easy
medium
hard

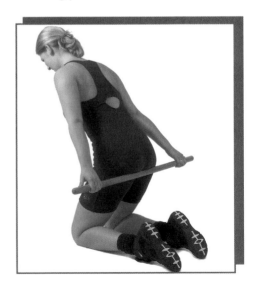

100 Strengthening exercise with a bar

TRAINING GOAL   **Strengthening** the abdominal muscles

Description
Starting position: Take up the "basic supine position". Grip the bar in front of your chest.

Exercise: Push the ends of the bar together, pushing your arms out to the sides.

Tips
- Keep your cervical spine straight; look upwards.
- Raise your shoulder blades clearly from the floor. Aim to move your sternum upwards.

Variation
a. Change the grip.

difficulty
easy
medium
hard

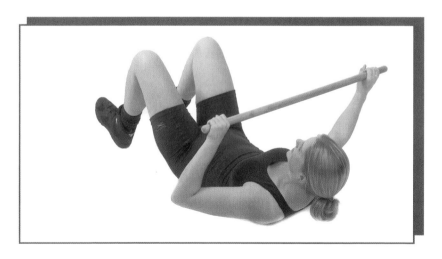

101 Strengthening exercise with a bar

Training Goal   **Strengthening** the stomach muscles

Description
Starting position: Take up the "basic supine position". Raise your legs at right angles to the floor. Grip the bar from below, under your legs.
Exercise: Extend your cervical spine and shoulder girdle. Push the ends of the bar together.

Tips
■■ Try to move your sternum upwards, consciously keeping your cervical spine extended.
■■ The bar should not touch the back of your thighs.

Variationen
a. Pull at the ends of the bar.
b. Alternate putting up your legs together and/or seperately.

difficulty
easy
medium
hard

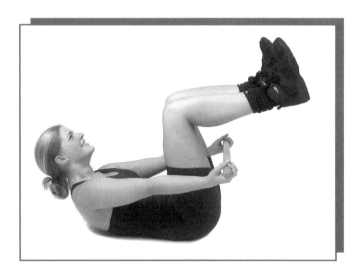

102 Strengthening exercise with a bar

Training Goal Strengthening the abdominal muscles

Description
Starting position: Take up the "basic supine position". Hold the bar in a u-position behind your head.

Exercise: Stretch your thoracic spine starting at your head as far as your shoulder blades.
Keep your arms off the floor and pull the ends of the bar apart. Lie back down on the floor again and push the ends of the bar together.

Tips
■ Look upwards rather than forwards. Do not make a "double chin".
■ Your lumbar spine remains on the floor.

Variation
a. In addition, raise your legs from the floor and extend them diagonally forwards and upwards.

difficulty
easy
medium
hard

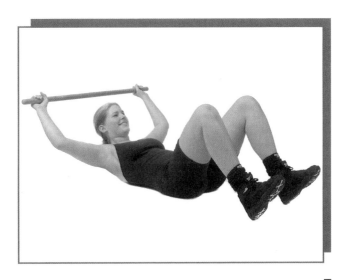

103 Strengthening exercise with a bar and a partner

TRAINING GOAL   **Strengthening** the oblique abdominal muscles
Stabilising the whole trunk

Exercise situation: Both partners carry out the same exercise together.

Description
Starting position: Stand up straight next to each other.
Hold the bar with the hand nearest your partner at stomach height.
Exercise: Pull the bar out to the side, without twisting your torso.

Tips
■■ Keep your spine stable by tensing your lower trunk muscles.

Variation
a. Carry out the exercise with the bar at shoulder height.

difficulty
easy
medium
hard

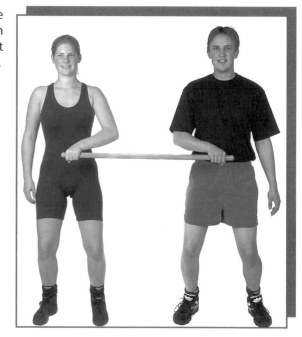

104 Strengthening exercise with a bar

TRAINING GOAL   **Strengthening** the shoulder girdle muscles
Strengthening the front thigh muscles

Description
Starting position: Stand up straight with your feet shoulder-width apart. Hold the bar vertically with both hands behind your back.
Exercise: Bend your knees and slide your hands down the bar. Finally bring the hands slowly back up to the top of the bar and stand up straight again.

Tips
- ▬ Keep your feet flat on the floor.
- ▬ Bend your knees no further than right angles.
- ▬ Keep your upper body almost vertical.

Variation
a. As described, now hold the bar in front of your body.

difficulty
easy
medium
hard

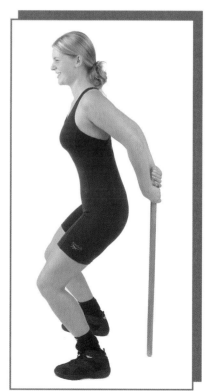

105 Strengthening exercise with a bar and a partner

TRAINING GOAL **Strengthening** the front thigh muscles
Awareness of the upright spinal posture

Exercise situation: Both partners carry out the same exercise together.

Description
Starting position: Stand opposite your partner with your feet shoulder-width apart with your legs slightly bent, holding the bar between you. Both upper bodies lean slightly backwards.

Exercise: Slowly bend your knees maximally until they are at right angles and then slowly straighten them again.

Tips
■ Tense your stomach and buttock muscles to stabilize your torso and push your pelvis forward slightly.
■ Your arms should hardly move.
■ Place your toes close together.

Variations
a. While one partner stands up straight, the other moves downwards. Maintain the tension between you!
b. Carry out the exercise holding 2 bars parallel between you.
c. Vary the grip: hold the bar from below and from above.

difficulty
easy
medium
hard

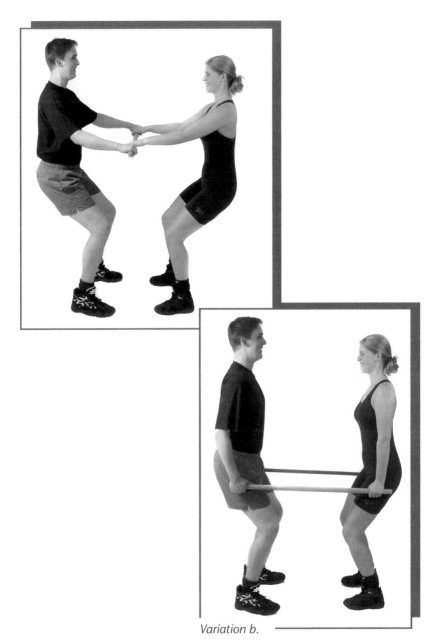

Variation b.

VI Relaxation Exercise –
Spoil Yourself at the End

106 Relaxation exercise

Description
Lay on your back. Make yourself as comfortable as possible. Remove everything from your mind that could disturb your relaxation. If necessary, fetch a cushion or a blanket; take off your shoes:

"Close your eyes and breathe in deeply, then breathe out slowly. Then start concentrating on breathing deeply, calmly and evenly from your stomach.

Breathe away more tension each time you exhale. Feel as though you are sinking deeper and deeper into the floor, relaxing and letting go more and more.

All of your tension should flow off into the floor.

Relax your eye muscles. Feel how your face relaxes, your forehead becomes smooth and unwrinkled, feel your scalp relax.

Your jaw relaxes and your teeth move apart, a certain cramping and crossness from stress and tension disappears, replaced by a feeling of relaxation in your face and your whole body.

Interiorise more and more how calmly and evenly you breathe and how relaxed this makes you feel. Feel how calm and composed and well balanced you become – each breath increases your feeling of wellbeing.

How does your back feel?
Direct your thoughts to your back for a moment.
Your back relaxes.
Your back muscles loosen.
Breathe once consciously in your back. What do you feel?
Your back becomes warm and relaxed.
Your back becomes heavy.
The skin on your back becomes smooth and relaxed.
Your back becomes heavy.
Your shoulder girdle, your shoulder blades press into the floor, your buttocks and pelvis too.

Your lumbar spine sinks relaxed into the floor.
Your whole body feels heavy.
You are completely calm, relaxed and composed.
Enjoy your relaxation."

Revoke your relaxation with a small tensing and moving exercise.

Tips
■ Trust the relaxing feeling of the exercise. Let yourself go. You have control over yourself at all times and can stop the exercise whenever you want.
■ With the concentration on breathing and on your back, this exercise develops the relaxation of your whole body.
■ To start with, focus on your breathing. A calm and regular breathing from your stomach for 3-5 minutes leads to good relaxation for your body and your spirit. With a conscious adoption of the exercise procedure, you will very easily transfer the effects to your soul.

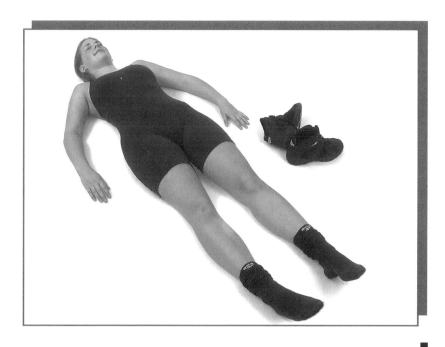

175

Bibliography

AHLAND, A.: Neuromuskuläre Kraftlenkung in der Haltungsschulung. Stuttgart 1996.

BOECKH-BEHRENS, W.-U./ BUSKIES, W.: Gesundheitsorientiertes Fitnesstraining. Band 1. 2. Auflage. Lüneburg 1996.

JORDAN, A.: Entspannungstraining. Ruhe für Körper, Geist und Seele. Aachen 1997.

JORDAN, A.: Fitness mit dem Thera-Band. Teil 1. In: Betrifft Sport 19 (1997) 1, 30-38.

JORDAN, A./GRAEBER, I.: Fitness zu zweit. Partnergymnastik – Dehnen und Kräftigen. Aachen 2000.

JORDAN, A./HILLEBRECHT, M.: Gymnastik mit dem Pezziball. Übungsprogramme. 3. Auflage. Aachen 1997.

JORDAN, A./HILLEBRECHT, M.: Gesundheitstraining mit dem Fit-Ball. Kräftigen – Dehnen – Entspannen. 2. Auflage. Aachen 1998.

KEMPF, H.-D.: Die Rückenschule. Das ganzheitliche Programm für einen gesunden Rücken. Reinbek 1995.

KEMPF, H.-D./SCHMELCHER, F./ZIEGLER, C.: Trainingsbuch Rückenschule. Reinbek 1996.

KOSCHEL, D./FERIÉ, C.: Vorbeugende Wirbelsäulen-Gymnastik. Aachen 1997.

MEDLER, M./MIELKE, W.: Rückenschule im Schulsport. Neumünster 1994.

MICHAELIS, P.: Moderne funktionelle Gymnastik. Aachen 2000.

REICHARDT, H.: Das ist Schongymnastik. Der gesunde Weg zu Beweglichkeit und Wohlbefinden. München 1993.

RÖßLER, S.: Krankengymnastische Gruppenbehandlung – mit Pfiff. 2. Auflage. Stuttgart, Jena, New York 1993.

SCHMIDT, N./HILLEBRECHT, M.: Übungsprogramme zur Dehn- und Kräftigungsgymnastik. Aachen 1992.

SCHMIDT, N./HILLEBRECHT, M.: Übungsprogramme zur Rücken- und Rumpfgymnastik. Aachen 1993.

Photo & Illustrations Credits

Cover photo: Engel-Korus, Know How für Sport, Fitness und Gesundheit, Ingelheim
Photos: Rudolf Hillebrecht
Cover design: Birgit Engelen